OPHTHALMOLOGY

MODERN NURSING SERIES

General Editors

A. J. HARDING RAINS, M.S., F.R.C.S.
Professor of Surgery, Charing Cross Hospital Medical School, University of London; Honorary Consultant Surgeon, Charing Cross Hospital; Honorary Consultant Surgeon to the Army.
VALERIE HUNT, S.R.N., S.C.M., O.N.D., R.N.T.
District Nursing Officer, Southmead Health District, Avon Area Health Authority, (Teaching), past Chairman General Nursing Council of England and Wales.

A SELECTION OF TITLES AVAILABLE AS PAPERBACKS

Psychology and Psychiatry for Nurses
PETER J. DALLY, M.B., F.R.C.P., D.P.M.
HEATHER HARRINGTON, S.R.N., R.M.N.

Community Health and Social Services
J. B. MEREDITH DAVIES, M.D., F.F.C.M., D.P.H.

Sociology in Nursing
R. KENNETH JONES, B.A., Ph.D., A.C.E.
PATRICIA JONES, S.R.N.

Neurology
EDWIN R. BICKERSTAFF, M.D., M.R.C.P.

Therapeutics
J. G. LEWIS, M.D., F.R.C.P.

Physiology for Nurses
DERYCK TAVERNER, M.B.E., M.D., F.R.C.P.

The Older Patient
a textbook of geriatrics
R. E. IRVINE, M.A., M.D., F.R.C.P.
M. K. BAGNALL, A.I.M.S.W.
B. J. SMITH, S.R.N., R.F.N.

Emergency and Acute Care
A. J. HARDING RAINS, M.S., F.R.C.S.
KEITH W. REYNOLDS, M.S., F.R.C.S.
VALERIE HUNT, S.R.N., S.C.M., O.N.D., R.N.T.

Ear, Nose and Throat Surgery and Nursing
R. PRACY, M.B., B.S., F.R.C.S.
J. SIEGLER, M.B., B.S., D.L.O., F.R.C.S.
P. M. STELL, M.B., F.R.C.S., A.I.L.
J. ROGERS, M.A., F.R.C.S.

Microbiology in Patient Care
H. I. WINNER, M.D., F.R.C.P., F.R.C.Path.

Textbook of Medicine
with relevant physiology and anatomy
R. J. HARRISON, Ch.B., M.D.

OPHTHALMOLOGY

IAN M. DUGUID

M.D., Ph.D., F.R.C.S., D.O.

Consultant Surgeon, Moorfields Eye Hospital, London
Ophthalmic Surgeon, Westminster Hospital, London

ANNE A. BERRY

S.R.N., O.N.D., BTA Cert., C.M.B. Part I. Middle Management Cert.

Area Nurse Health Care Services Planning,
Kent Area Health Authority

HODDER AND STOUGHTON

LONDON SYDNEY AUCKLAND TORONTO

ISBN 0 340 05207 4 Boards
ISBN 0 340 05206 6 Paperback

First printed 1971
Reprinted with additions 1975
Reprinted 1978

Printed and bound in Great Britain for
Hodder and Stoughton Educational,
a division of Hodder and Stoughton Ltd,
Mill Road, Dunton Green, Sevenoaks, Kent,
by Biddles Ltd, Guildford, Surrey

EDITOR'S FOREWORD

This book is related to a series of textbooks written specially for students of nursing, midwifery, physiotherapy, speech training and medical social work. The series is designed to cover the requirements of the State Registration Examinations conducted by the General Nursing Council. Where appropriate, each book is written by a physician or a surgeon in conjunction with a sister tutor or nursing tutor. This is with the deliberate intention of stressing the close association between clinical medicine and nursing.

Diseases of the eye merit a degree of meticulous attention to the examination and care of patients. The authors, one a distinguished consultant ophthalmic surgeon, the other Assistant Matron at the Western Ophthalmic Hospital, both have long experience in the training of ophthalmic nursing students. It is to these students that this book is primarily addressed. However, a handy book of explanation of the practice of ophthalmic medicine and surgery is in demand for the general medical and nursing staffs in the very centres of hospital service, in the clinic, the ward, the operating theatre and in the casualty department. I am confident that this book will long fill the general as well as the specialist need.

A. J. Harding Rains

PREFACE

This book has been written concisely and explicitly to provide accounts of ocular disorders suitable for instructing nurses in the first instance, but it is hoped that medical students may also find the book of value while newly graduated doctors might also utilise it as a handy reference. This book should cover the ground for nurses studying for their ophthalmic nursing diploma examinations.

Following an introductory chapter, disorders of the eyeball and its adnexa have been divided into easily assimilated sections, while this is followed by a section indicating nursing procedures primarily designed to help nurses with treatments.

Unfortunately, it has been necessary to reduce illustrations in number but it is hoped that this will not be a detraction.

We acknowledge our thanks to Dr. P. Hansell, Director of the Audiovisual Department, Institute of Ophthalmology for preparing the illustrations and to Mr T. Tarrant of the same department for his excellent diagrams. The chapter on strabismus has been the work of Miss Ann Hughes, D.B.O.(T.) of Moorfields Eye Hospital, High Holborn, London and further appreciation is due to Baillière, Tindall and Cassell for Fig. 13. from Wybar's *Ophthalmology*. Messrs C. Davis Keeler have kindly donated Figs. 2 – 5 together with Plates 8 and 9.

Finally, Mr M. S. Davies willingly read over the text and suggested many useful amendments incorporated in various chapters while Dr. D. J. Darby kindly prepared the Index. The burden of secretarial assistance has been carried by Mrs Doreen Stiles and to a lesser extent by Miss Helen Inman. We should like also to express appreciation for the help and encouragement received from the Editorial Staff of The English Universities Press Ltd.

I. M. Duguid
A. A. Berry

CONTENTS

1 *EXAMINATION OF THE EYE*

INTRODUCTION

Prior to an examination of the eyes it is essential that a careful history is taken. The exact onset and nature of the complaint should be noted, while the occurrence of any eye trouble in the family pedigree should not be omitted. Particular questioning should also be made about vision, pain in and around the eyes, watering and discharge from the eyes, as clues about the aetiology of an eye disorder are sometimes revealed in the history.

Examination of the eye may be considered in two parts: (1) objective examination and (2) subjective examination.

1 OBJECTIVE EXAMINATION

Objective examination of the ocular appendages and anterior parts of the eyeball is by inspection and palpation. Inspection entails the observation of any redness, discharge, lacrimation, obvious squint and any undue prominences or distortion of the eyes and/or eyelids. The inner aspects of both upper and lower lids are examined.

Next, the eyeball movements should be ascertained and note be made of abnormal position and excursion.

Sometimes the conjunctiva becomes congested (i.e. injected), oedematous (chemosis) or even discoloured.

Corneal examination follows, and it is important to examine the integrity of its epithelium by instilling 2% fluorescein solution or 1% Bengal Rose, preferably one or two drops, and the excess is washed away with sterile normal (0·9%) saline or water. With fluorescein absence of corneal epithelium shows a green coloration corresponding with the defect whereas intact epithelium shows no staining. Diseased cornea is usually opacified; if only slightly so, the opacity is called a *nebula* while a denser scar is referred to as a *leucoma.*

A wisp of cotton wool is frequently used to test corneal sensitivity but more refined tests may be utilised if need be.

The depth and clarity of the anterior chamber should be examined together with its contained aqueous humour. Normal, average or deep are terms commonly used to designate the former, while normal aqueous humour is clear; in pathological states, it becomes hazy and even contains exudate which, if dense, presents as a yellow deposit of pus (hypopyon). Sometimes, blood appears in the anterior chamber (hyphaema). Like the cornea, it is necessary to examine the anterior chamber with a fine strong light to demonstrate cells in the aqueous which may be deposited on the interior of the cornea (keratic precipitates or K.P.).

Healthy iris is blue or brown with several intermediate variations, but diseased iris often undergoes an alteration in colour while its contour may become ill-defined and new vessel formation (rubeosis) appears on its surface. Adhesions of

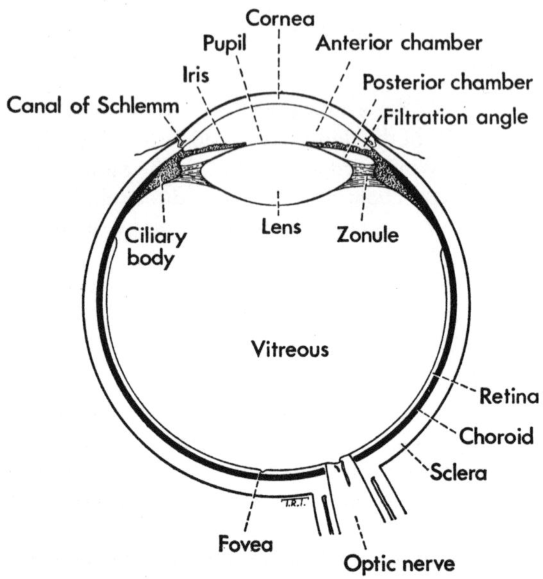

FIG 1 Horizontal section of the eye

iris to cornea are referred to as anterior synechiae, and posterior synechiae are adhesions between iris and lens but they may be between iris and vitreous, e.g. after lens extraction. Support to the iris is generally given by the lens but when the lens is displaced or absent the iris becomes tremulous (iridodonesis).

The size, shape and position of the pupil should be noted. In addition its reaction to light and accommodation are observed. The pupil size tends to be in a constant state of flux (hippus).

The normal lens is transparent but deposits may appear on the surface or within the lens (cataract). The ophthalmoscope and/or slit lamp are used for examination of the lens, vitreous and fundus, an inspection usually performed by ophthalmologists.

Palpation may be utilised for examination of the lids, particularly if lid cysts or tumours are suspected, while palpation of the globe may elicit tenderness of the eye itself as in inflammations involving the uveal tract. In addition palpation of the eye, using the index fingers, will give a *rough* indication of the intraocular tension, for example, if it is raised, about normal or lower. However, for more refined measurement of the intraocular tension a tonometer is used: the Schiötz tonometer is in most general use but the applanation tonometer now replaces it in many clinics. For tonometry two drops of 1% amethocaine are instilled and the patient lies down on a couch for the recording to be made by Schiötz tonometer. The Schiötz tonometer is then placed on the cornea of the widely opened eye and the tonometer needle or pointer is deflected along the scale. This deflection is noted and the accompanying chart translates it into millimetres of mercury. A normal tension is below 25 mm of mercury as registered by Schiötz tonometer, while raised tension lies above this level. Palpation may be of value in detecting abnormalities e.g. fracture of the orbital margin and sometimes tumours in the anterior orbit may even be felt. (See page 110 and Plate 12.)

2 SUBJECTIVE EXAMINATION

The testing of the function of each eye separately is dependent upon the statements of the patient. The functions tested are the form sense, the fields of vision, the colour sense and the light sense.

Visual Acuity

Acuity of vision is the expression of form sense, which is the faculty each eye has of perceiving the shape of objects. This acuity is tested both for distant and near vision.

Distant Vision

This is usually tested with the test-type set at 6 metres (20 ft) from the subject because rays of light from the point at this distance are almost parallel. Snellen's test-type, which is the type often used in testing, is constructed with each letter (Fig. 2) inscribed within a square which subtends a visual angle of 5′ at the distance at which the normal eye should distinguish the letter. The visual angle lies within

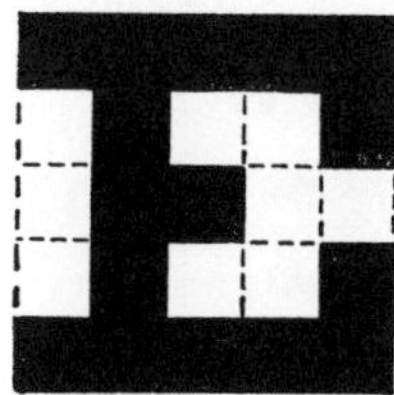

FIG 2 Construction of Snellen's test-type

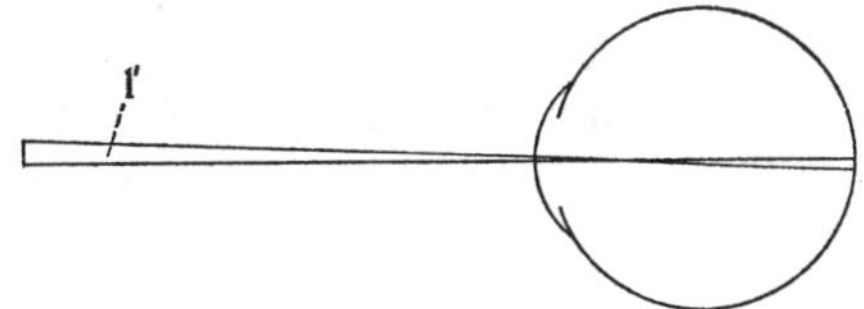

FIG 3 Minimum separable (1′ = angle of one minute at the nodal point)

two lines from the extremities of the object through the nodal point of the eye (Fig. 3). It will be seen (Fig. 2) that the square is made up of five smaller ones of equal size so that the smaller ones therefore subtend a visual angle of 1′. This is the minimum visual angle for a normal eye.

The square-shaped serif letters on the test-types decrease in size from above downwards on the chart (Fig. 4). The letters are of such a size that the normal eye

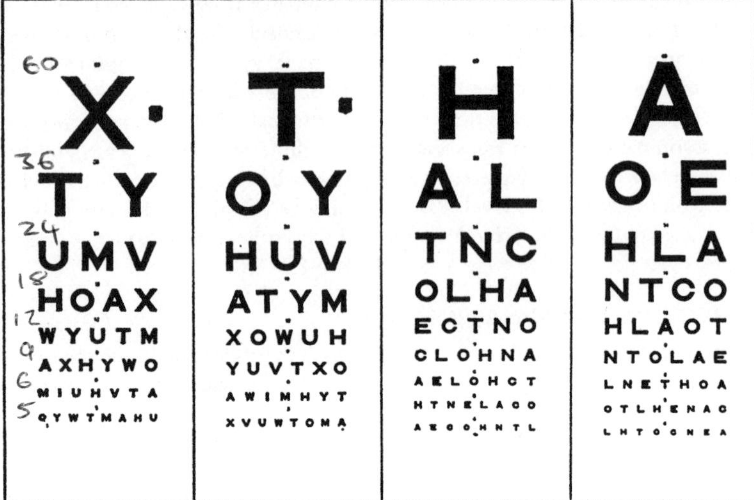

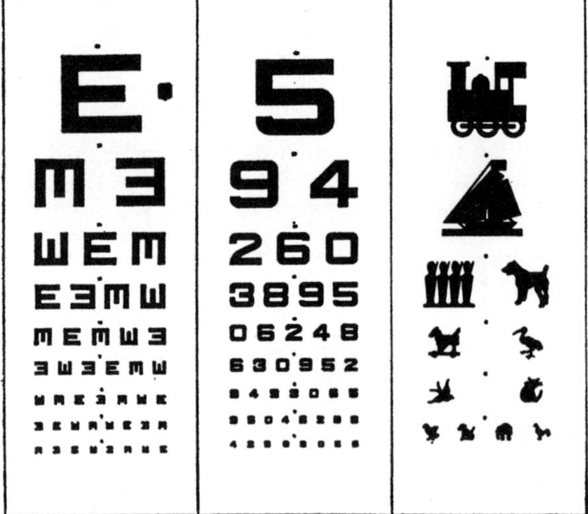

FIG 4 Test-types

should discern the top one at 60 metres, while the following rows should be read by the normal eye at 36, 24, 18, 12, 9, 6 and 5 metres respectively. As it is impracticable to see the type at these distances, it is usually placed 6 metres in front of the patient. The visual acuity is expressed as a fraction, the numerator signifying the distance of the patient from the chart e.g. 6 metres, and the denominator the number indicating the distance at which the lowest or smallest row of letters is read by the normal eye. A patient with normal vision should, 6 metres away from the chart, read the second lowest line on the chart (Fig. 4) and have his vision recorded as 6/6. On the other hand if a patient only perceives the fourth line on the chart, the visual acuity of this eye under test is 6/18. If the patient is unable to read the top letter on the chart, the distance is reduced. If he recognises the top letter at 3 metres, the visual acuity is 3/60. If he cannot read the top letter at any distance, he is asked to count fingers held against a dark background: perception of the fingers at 3 m is recorded as counts fingers (C.F.) at 3 m. Sometimes, the visual acuity is reduced even further and the patient may only recognise hand movements at 1 or 2 m and then we note it as H.M. at 1 m or H.M. at 2 m. With an even greater reduction of vision, light is shone on the eye and we ascertain if there is perception of light (P.L.).

Ideally, the test-type should be evenly illuminated, the chart should be about the level of the patient's eyes and the patient should have his back to any window(s). The vision of each eye is separately tested.

For children and illiterate patients, the 'E' test may be used and the subject is given a wooden 'E' which he holds in the same position as the one on the test-type being pointed to by the examiner. Landolt's rings may be used as an alternative or variant of the 'E' test.

Near Vision

For proper focusing of divergent rays from a near point, an increase in refractive power of the eye (accommodation) is required. The type utilised for near vision testing consists of ordinary printer's types of different sizes (Fig. 5). A normal patient should be able to read the smallest type about 33 cm away with each eye.

Field of Vision

The field of vision is the term used to indicate the representation of the limits of peripheral vision i.e. the extent of limits of what one sees. This may be charted by *confrontation* but a more accurate estimation of the peripheral visual fields may be obtained by use of the *perimeter* (Plate 9).

A defect in the visual field, scotoma, may also be charted using a Bjerrum screen. The screen, usually black or grey, is fixed on a wall and the patient situated one or two metres from the screen. The field is charted for about 30° around fixation.

Colour Sense

Colour vision may be tested using a colour lantern, of which the Edridge Green is probably best known and which emits light of different colours. In addition to the lantern test, coloured plates (Ishihara) are frequently used. A further variant is the coloured wool test which depends on the discrimination of wool of different colours.

N. 5

He moved forward a few steps; the house was so dark behind him, the world so dim and uncertain in front of him, that for a moment his heart failed him. He might have to search the whole garden for the dog. Then he heard a sniff, felt something wet against his leg—he had almost stepped upon the animal. He bent down and stroked its wet coat. The dog stood quite still, then moved forward towards the house, sniffed at the steps, at last walked calmly through the open door as though the house belonged to him. Jeremy followed, closed the door behind them; then there they were in the little dark passage with the boy's heart beating like a drum, his teeth chattering, and a terrible temptation to sneeze hovering around him. Let him reach the nursery and establish the animal there and all might be well, but let them be discovered, cold and shivering, in the passage, and out the dog would be flung. He knew so exactly what would happen.

(From "Jeremy" by Hugh Walpole).

wire sons vain error unwise cream remove

N. 6

The camp stood where, until quite lately, had been pasture and ploughland; the farm house still stood in a fold of the hill and had served us for battalion offices; ivy still supported part of what had once been the walls of a fruit garden; half an acre of mutilated old trees behind the wash-houses survived of an orchard. The place had been marked for destruction before the army came to it. Had there been another year of peace, there would have been no farmhouse, no wall, no apple trees. Already half a mile of concrete road lay between bare clay banks, and on either side a chequer of open ditches showed where the municipal contractors had designed a system of drainage. Another year of peace would have made the place part of the neighbouring suburb. Now the huts where we had wintered waited their turn for destruction.

(From " Brideshead Revisited " by Evelyn Waugh)

nervous manner immune over unanimous wear

N. 8

And another image came to me, of an arctic hut and a trapper alone with his furs and oil lamp and log fire; the remains of supper on the table, a few books, skis in the corner; everything dry and neat and warm inside and outside the last blizzard of winter raging and the snow piling up against the door. Quite silently a great weight forming against the timber; the bolt straining in its socket; minute by minute in the darkness outside the white heap sealing the door, until quite soon when the wind dropped and the sun came out on the ice slopes and the thaw set in a block would move, slide and tumble high above, gather way, gather weight, till the whole hillside seemed to be falling, and the little lighted place would crash open and splinter and disappear, rolling with the avalanche into the ravine. ***(From " Brideshead Revisited " by Evelyn Waugh)***

immense snow came near arrow use.

FIG 5 Printer's test-types of different sizes

Light Sense

This entails the detection of light of different intensities, and the apparatus used for this is known as an adaptometer or photometer.

Refraction of the Eye

The refracting structures of the eye i.e. the cornea and lens and the axial length of the eye, are the factors upon which the refraction of the eye is dependent. Estimation of the refraction of the eye is dependent upon these factors, and its assessment enables one to determine the corrected visual acuity.

Refraction takes place when rays of light in one medium meet another of different optical density as, for example, when rays in air traverse the cornea. At the interface, the rays are bent from their original direction. This is illustrated in Fig. 6.

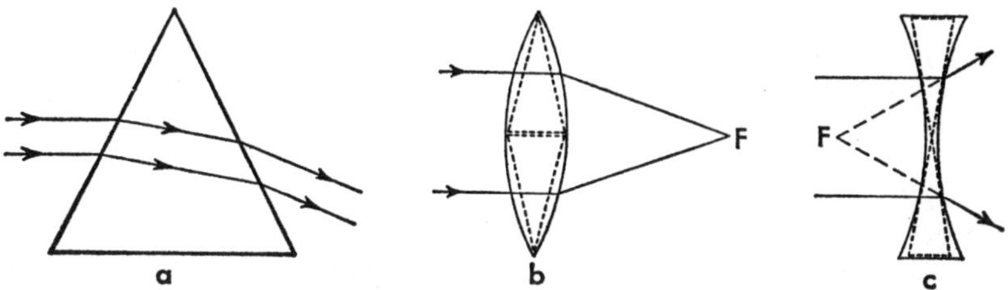

FIG 6 (a) Passage of light through a prism
(b) Convergence of parallel rays by a convex lens
(c) Divergence of parallel rays by a concave lens

(a) *The Cornea*

The most important refraction in the eye takes place at its anterior surface. This is because the cornea is more optically dense than the air in contact with it. In contrast, little refraction takes place at the interface between cornea and aqueous. The convex anterior surface of the cornea causes convergence of parallel incident rays, but at the posterior corneal surface the convergence is negligible.

(b) *The Lens*

The absence of any appreciable differences in optical densities between the lens and the surrounding media reduces the convergence of incident rays at these interfaces as compared with the convergence at the anterior corneal surface. However, there is an increase in the optical density of the centre of the lens (nucleus) while the periphery of the lens (cortex) is less optically dense. Furthermore, the lens may alter its refractivity by an alteration in shape. For example, an increase occurs in accommodation when the eye fixates on a near point.

(c) *Axial Length of the Eye*

Consideration of the axial length of the eye is essential in the determination of the refraction of the eye.

Rays of light emerging from the far point (punctum remotum) at infinity are parallel. These parallel rays enter an eye with normal refraction and are brought to a focus on the retina i.e. the eye is emmetropic. This condition (*emmetropia*) demands an exact correspondence between the axial length of the eye and the dioptric power of the ocular refracting media (Fig. 7).

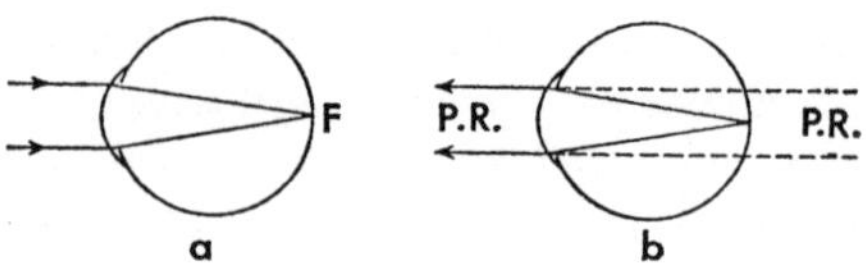

FIG 7 Refraction by the emmetropic eye

Ametropia

When parallel rays of light enter the eye and do not come to a focus on the retina *ametropia* is present. Ametropia exists in four different forms: (1) Hypermetropia (2) Myopia (3) Astigmatism (4) Anisometropia.

(1) *Hypermetropia*

In hypermetropia, parallel rays of light entering the eye would come to a focus behind the retina. This may be because the axial length of the eye is too short (axial hypermetropia) or because of a failure of the refracting media to bring the rays to a focus on the retina e.g. decreased density. Usually, the hypermetropic eye is smaller than the normal. When the hypermetropia is not corrected by lenses an extra effort must be made to maintain accommodation and thereby a clear image; this effort may give rise to eye strain while in young children squint may sometimes be a sequel. Convex correcting lenses are used to obtain a clear focus (Figs. 8 and 9).

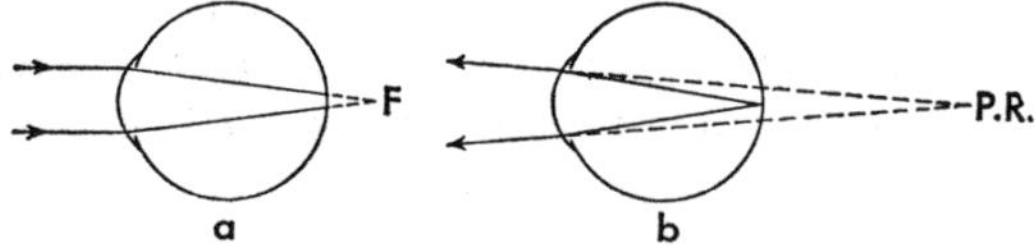

FIG 8 Refraction by the hypermetropic eye

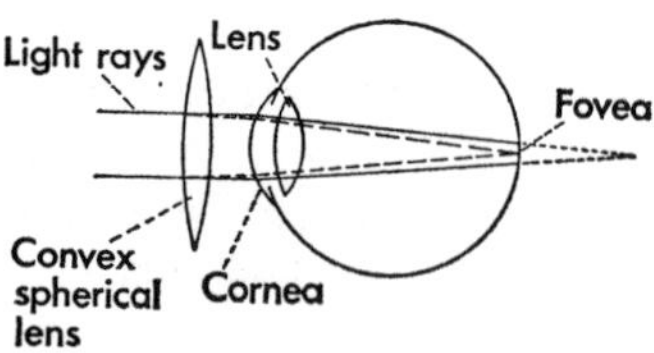

FIG 9 Correction of hypermetropia by a convex lens

(2) *Myopia*

In myopia, parallel rays of light entering the eye come to a focus in front of the retina. Myopia may be present when the axial length of the eye is greater than normal, when there is excessive corneal or lenticular curvature, or increased density of the nucleus of the lens. The myopic eye is usually larger than normal and enlargement involving the posterior part of the eye usually is visible with the ophthalmoscope when atrophy along the temporal border of the optic disc (myopic crescent) is present. In high myopia, the scleral thinning is marked and the ocular contents may even bulge backwards to give a posterior staphyloma.

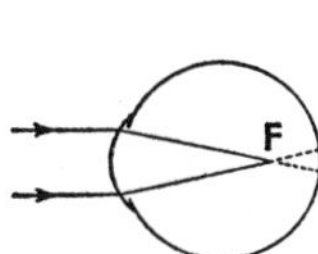

FIG 10 Refraction of the myopic eye

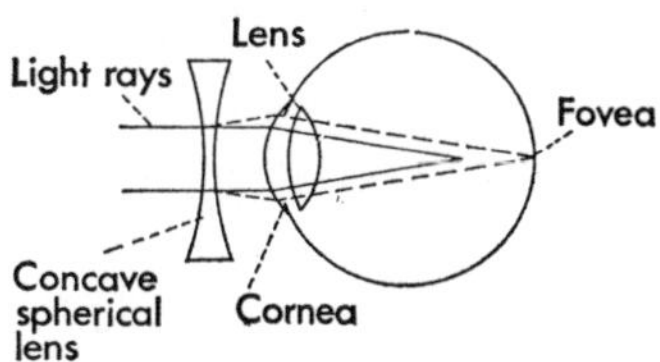

FIG 11 Correction of myopia by a concave lens

(3) *Astigmatism*

In astigmatism, parallel rays of light are not brought to a focus at the same point in all meridia. Astigmatism may be associated with hypermetropia when it is referred to as hypermetropic astigmatism, with myopia as myopic astigmatism or mixed astigmatism when one meridian is hypermetropic and the other myopic.

(4) *Anisometropia*

When there are unequal amounts of ametropia in each eye, anisometropia exists. Refraction may be measured by retinoscopy or by correcting lenses.

In hypermetropia, convex lenses are used to obtain convergence of incident parallel rays of light so that they then approximate each other, and come to a focus on the retina. On the other hand, in myopia concave lenses are utilised so that parallel rays of light are made to diverge and focus on the retina instead of in front of it.

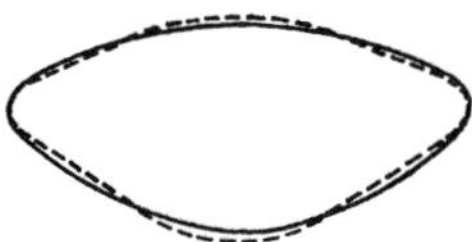

FIG 12 Changes in shape of lens with accommodation (dotted line) and when relaxed (continuous line)

As a person ages, his ability to focus on near objects lessens because the lens of the eye less readily alters shape in response to the stimulus for accommodation. Such an inability produces a blurred image for near objects—*presbyopia*. Presbyopia usually has its onset about the age of 45 years when a convex lens of +0·5 sphere is added to the corrected distant vision in order to obtain clarity of near print or objects, while the required strength of the convex lens increases as one approaches 60 years of age till +3·0 sphere may be needed.

Most refractive errors are corrected by spectacle lenses but contact lenses are becoming more popular, particularly in the correction of myopia. Contact lenses fit on the anterior corneal surface and eliminate its refractive influence.

2 *DISEASES OF THE EYELIDS*

ANATOMY

The eyelids, upper and lower, are both mobile and help to protect the eyeballs. Superficially, they are covered by thin skin which merges at the intermarginal strip (or free border) with the conjunctiva lining the deep surface of the lid. From the anterior border of the free border project two or three rows of lashes or cilia. A layer of connective tissue lies below the skin separating it from muscle, the orbicularis oculi, and, in the upper lid, the levator palpebrae superioris. The orbicularis oculi is supplied by the seventh cranial nerve (facial nerve) and forms a flattened band of concentric fibres surrounding the opening between the lids (palpebral aperture). The muscle is thus ideally suited for closing the lids but it also aids drainage of tears along the lacrimal canaliculi to the lacrimal sac and nasolacrimal duct. The levator palpebrae superioris arises from the apex of the orbit, passes forwards below the roof of the orbit to the orbital margin, when it passes inferiorly into the upper lid to be inserted into the tarsal plate to the skin of the lid and to the middle of the lateral and medial orbital margins. The tarsal plate lies between the orbicularis muscle fibres superficially and the conjunctiva on its deep aspect. The tarsal plate is composed of dense fibrous tissue which is prolonged medially and laterally to gain their respective attachments to the medial and lateral orbital margins. These prolongations are known as the medial and lateral palpebral ligaments which contribute towards the maintenance of the acutely angled outer part of the palpebral aperture (lateral canthus) and towards the elliptical medial part (medial canthus) of the aperture.

Situated in the tarsal plate are about 20–40 tarsal or meibomian glands, running vertically in the lids and opening via fine ductules onto the posterior part of the intermarginal strip of the lids. These glands are modified sebaceous glands whose secretions help to prevent overflowing of tears from the conjunctival sac. In addition to the openings of the tarsal glands in the intermarginal portion of the lid, there are the openings of lacrimal canaliculi. These openings are known as the lacrimal puncta; one punctum is situated on each lid about 6–8 mm from the inner canthus.

With the eyes directed straight forwards and the eyelids normally opened, the margin of the lower lid is at the same level as the corneo-scleral junction, but the level of the margin of the upper lid encroaches upon the cornea for about 2 mm.

CONGENITAL ABNORMALITIES

Coloboma

This developmental anomaly is a defect or notching of the eyelid margin of variable extent and usually situated at the junction of the inner and middle thirds of the upper eyelid. The notch may be sufficiently large to give exposure of the cornea. It is then necessary to close the defect by plastic surgery, thereby protecting the cornea.

Epicanthus

This is a crescentic fold of skin which partly obscures the medial canthus as it stretches from the medial part of the eyebrow to the lower lid. Its prominence varies and it is usually bilateral, but it is particularly evident in the Mongolian race. Epicanthic folds tend to disappear spontaneously as the bridge of the nose develops but, while the folds are present, a convergent strabismus may be thought to be present (pseudo strabismus) when no actual strabismus exists. Marked epicanthic folds may be found with a congenital ptosis and narrowing of the palpebral aperture (blepharophimosis).

Distichiasis

Distichiasis is an anomaly involving one or both lids in whole or part, and in which an extra row of eyelashes is present.

Ptosis

The name given to a drooping of the upper eyelid is ptosis. It may be unilateral or bilateral, and occurs as a congenital anomaly due to defective development of the levator palpebrae superioris. This anomaly may also be associated with weakness of the superior rectus muscle of the eye. The degree of drooping varies between patients but, if excessive, the lid constantly encroaches on the pupil and thereby prevents normal visual function. Surgical correction will diminish the ptosis but no surgery is needed for minor degrees of ptosis. Elevation of a ptotic lid may also be obtained by ptosis props attached to spectacle frames.

Ankyloblepharon

Adhesion between the upper and lower eyelids is known as ankyloblepharon. The area of union between the lids varies greatly in extent but the adhesion may be readily treated by simple division.

Lagophthalmos

Incomplete closure of the palpebral aperture when the eyelids are shut may result as a congenital anomaly. The importance of the condition lies in the resultant exposure of the eyeball (see page 72).

INFLAMMATIONS INVOLVING THE EYELIDS

Blepharitis

This is a chronic inflammation involving the margins of the eyelids. It is traditional to look upon it as existing in two forms: (1) Squamous (non-ulcerative) and (2) Ulcerative.

Squamous blepharitis is characterised by redness and some swelling of the lid margins together with the accumulation of yellowish white, scaly deposits on the eyelashes. Removal of these scales may reveal small ulcers (ulcerative blepharitis) which readily bleed and which may be accompanied by loss of eyelashes. Continuing infection gives rise to distortion of the lashes which turn inwards (trichiasis) to irritate the eyeball. A seborrhoeic dermatitis is frequently present with squamous blepharitis which itself has an increased incidence in childhood and adolescence.

TREATMENT

All scales must be removed daily from the lid margins. This is most easily done using cotton-wool moistened in warm water. Once these scales are removed, application of antibiotic ointment e.g. oculentum neomycin is beneficial. Further relief is obtained by incorporating cortisone in the oculentum, while a medicated shampoo for the scalp is also of value. Attention to hygiene and improvement of general health has also been advocated, but it is doubtful if the correction of refractive errors is helpful. Electrolysis of the ingrowing lashes destroys them and is often preferable to recurrent epilation of the offending lashes. Unfortunately, treatment is usually long drawn out because its cessation is accompanied by a return of the blepharitis.

Stye (External Hordeolum)

This is an inflammation of the lash follicle and is usually acute and painful. In most cases, oedema and redness at the site of the inflammation are evident while, in more advanced cases, yellow pus may also point there or even discharge from the follicle. Styes occur at all ages and also tend to appear in crops.

TREATMENT

The most effective is epilation of the lash; its removal allows drainage of pus within the infected follicle. Heat in the form of hot bathing or formentations has often been followed by relief.

Chalazion (Meibomian Cyst)

This results from an obstruction of the ductule of a meibomian gland. The sebaceous secretions from the gland accumulate while the gland enlarges to form a painless swelling which is usually found away from the lid margin. Infection may supervene amidst the stagnant secretions to give rise to redness and pain. Eversion of the eyelid shows a yellowish area with surrounding hyperaemia at the site of the chalazion. (Plate 1.)

TREATMENT

A small chalazion may subside spontaneously but surgery is usually necessary. The area around the chalazion, the conjunctiva, is anaesthetised by 1% guttae amethocaine or 4% guttae cocaine and the remaining tissues of the lid locally by lignocaine or procaine injected into the lid. The lid is then everted by a chalazion clamp applied around the cyst and the conjunctiva overlying the chalazion is incised and the contents evacuated by curettage. Incision and curettage through the skin can be done if pointing occurs superficially, while excision of the mass is necessary if fibrous replacement has occurred in the cyst. Systemic antibiotic is desirable in the presence of gross sepsis.

Sebaceous cysts may appear on the cutaneous surface of an eyelid. They are elevated, white and often of small size. Incision and curettage effect removal of the cyst contents.

Cyst of the Gland of Moll

This is a painless translucent enlargement of the gland situated on the skin of the eyelid near an eyelash which may be removed by cautery or excision.

Herpes Simplex

This is a viral eruption which presents on the eyelids but which is often coincident or associated with viral involvement elsewhere e.g. lips, nose and cornea.

Vaccinia

This results from the inoculation (usually accidental) of an eyelid with the virus from a smallpox vaccination. There is marked oedema and redness of the eyelid or eyelids together with enlargement of the preauricular and submaxillary lymph nodes. Regression is spontaneous in most cases but recovery may be accelerated by the intramuscular injection of gamma globulin.

Syphilis of the Eyelids

A primary chancre rarely occurs on the eyelids but when present often arises as a result of self-inoculation from a genital chancre. A regional adenitis is usual. In the secondary stage, skin rashes may involve the eyelids and gummatous tarsitis may occur in tertiary syphilis.

Herpes Zoster Ophthalmicus

Unilateral vesicular eruption, oedema, hyperaemia and impaired sensation characterise this condition, which involves the skin of the affected side of the face and scalp supplied by the ophthalmic division of the trigeminal nerve (fifth cranial nerve).

Patients suffering from this condition have previously suffered from chickenpox, albeit many years before. Pre-herpetic pain along the site of the eruption precedes the vesiculation and oedema by about three days. The vesicles become opalescent and purulent besides having a surrounding halo of injection before becoming crusted. Later, these crusts are shed wherever they may be along the distribution of the ophthalmic branch of the trigeminal nerve.

Fifty per cent of cases have involvement of the eyeball, which is reputedly more likely if the nasociliary nerve is involved. Injection and chemosis with or without corneal infiltration signify ocular complications, while iridocyclitis (with its inflammatory deposits (keratic precipitates or K.P.) on the corneal endothelium) may precipitate secondary glaucoma. Impaired or absent corneal sensation is evident, while paresis of the extrinsic ocular musculature rarely develops.

The cutaneous crusts are shed in two or three weeks but post-herpetic pain or neuralgia may persist for years.

Treatment consists of relief of the pain with analgesics and antibiotic ointment, calamine lotion, starch powder or bismuth powder are advocated for the cutaneous lesions. Atropine and cortisone drops are required not only for the keratitis but also for the iridocyclitis. When secondary glaucoma supervenes, the raised intraocular tension may have to be controlled by tabs. acetazolamide 250 mg once to thrice daily. One particularly trying complaint is the post-herpetic neuralgia pain, relief from which is very difficult to obtain.

Dermatitis

This may occur in conjunction with a generalised dermatitis but may also be localised to the eyelids. In the latter instance, it may be due to irritation from drugs applied to the eye. Atropine, penicillin, sulphonamides and eserine applied in drop forms are the most common causes, but the application of ointment can also cause irritation because of an allergy to the ointment base.

TUMOURS

Benign

(1) *Papilloma*

This is the most common tumour of the eyelids when it generally appears as a raised vascular pedunculated mass. Occasionally, it is flat and varying keratinisation on the surface gives it a horny appearance. It may be removed by simple excision.

(2) *Xanthelasma*

This is a slightly raised yellow tumour in the sebaceous glands, particularly those of the upper lid in its medial half. It also occurs in the lower lid. As it is unsightly, removal by simple excision may be indicated.

(3) *Angioma*

This abnormality of the blood vessels of the eyelids varies in colour from bright red (due to a capillary proliferation—telangiectasis) to a dark blue (due to an abnormal venous proliferation—cavernous angioma). Occasionally it forms part of a more extensive vascular tumour ('port wine' tumour) or it may even be associated with angiomata of the eyeball and brain (Sturge-Weber syndrome).

Angiomata are generally present at birth and become more prominent with crying or straining. Early treatment is contraindicated except when it does not permit adequate opening of the eyelids as they generally regress in size. Surgery may be contemplated for large unsightly ones while irradiation is sometimes also useful.

Malignant Tumours

(1) *Epithelioma*

This is a squamous-celled carcinoma of low malignancy. There is only a slight tendency to metastasise. Clinically, it usually presents on the eyelid margin as a small localised mass with a slightly raised margin and a liability to form a central ulcer. Treatment is surgical, which entails the excision of enough healthy surrounding tissue to ensure complete removal of the growth. As is the case in many carcinomata of the lids, excision of the tumour may have to be followed by plastic repair to make good the lid defect.

(2) *Basal-celled Carcinoma or Rodent Ulcer*

This tumour is most commonly situated towards the inner angle of the lower lid at its margin but may also be found in the skin around the eye. Clinically, it is nodular with a repeated tendency to form a crust which may break off and give a sero-sanguineous discharge. The local malignancy of the tumour is shown by extension of the mass from its periphery with invasion and destruction of surrounding tissue but little or no evidence of metastasis. Again, adequate surgical removal is the most satisfactory treatment although radiotherapy is sometimes indicated.

(3) *Malignant Melanoma*

This uncommon pigmented tumour of the eyelids may arise primarily in the tarsus or be metastatic. A blood-borne metastasis is more common than lymphatic spread.

3 *DISEASES OF THE CONJUNCTIVA*

ANATOMY

The conjunctiva is a mucous membrane which lines the internal aspect of the eyelids (palpebral or tarsal conjunctiva) from which it is reflected onto the anterior aspect of the eyeball (bulbar conjunctiva) as far as the limbus where it is continuous with the corneal epithelium. It forms small recesses where it is reflected from the upper and lower eyelids onto the eyeball: these are respectively called the superior and inferior fornix. The conjunctiva opens anteriorly between the margins of the two eyelids.

There is a profuse vascular network of arteries and veins coursing through the conjunctiva but many of these vessels are not readily visible because of their contraction. In addition to vessels, the conjunctiva contains both sensory nerve elements from the fifth cranial (trigeminal) nerve and glands (mucous and serous).

Furthermore, a crescentic fold of conjunctiva called the plica semilunaris lies near the inner canthus. Its lateral free border is directed towards the cornea. Medial to the plica is a red fleshy nodule of modified skin called the caruncle.

CONJUNCTIVITIS

Conjunctivitis is an inflammation of the conjunctiva which frequently occurs and which is usually infective (bacterial or viral) in origin, but it may also be allergic or associated with disorders of the skin.

Inflammatory

Normally, conjunctivitis is painless but discomfort, burning, grittiness, photophobia and excessive watering are common. Questioning often reveals a discharge from the eyes to be present, and this is often sufficient to cause the lids to be stuck together after sleep, but in lesser degrees of conjunctivitis only a mucoid or mucopurulent discharge is evident. The conjunctiva is red (injected), the colour being characteristically referred to as 'brick-red'. Although the conjunctival injection may be general, in some it is largely localised to the tarsal or to the bulbar conjunctiva; with bulbar injection, the conjunctiva may be freely moved over the surface of the eyeball. Accompanying the conjunctivitis is often some oedema of the conjunctiva (chemosis) while occasionally haemorrhage occurs subconjunctivally. Conjunctivitis occurs at all ages. (Plates 2 and 3.)

Varieties of Inflammatory Conjunctivitis

Purulent

This is usually caused by the *Neisseria gonorrhoea*, a Gram-negative diplococcus, which is found in abundant numbers within the purulent secretions. Newborn babies suffering from the condition are directly infected from a maternal genital infection which is transmitted to the baby's eyes during labour. It is rarely present in adults.

Incubation is usually short, varying from a few hours to three days. Profuse purulent discharge gathers within the red swollen lids which, when not tightly closed, emit a purulent discharge. The conjunctiva is heavily injected and infection may spread to involve the cornea when its epithelium is breached. The resultant corneal ulcer may quickly extend and corneal destruction gives perforation of the cornea with release of aqueous and incarceration of iris. Resolution at this stage produces *leucoma adherens* but when infection spreads an *endophthalmitis* results.

Treatment

Prophylactic: Cleansing of the lids with subsequent instillation of antibiotic (e.g. guttae sulphacetamide 10% or penicillin) after birth is indicated, but some still instil 1–2% silver nitrate as advocated by Crede during the 19th century. If only one eye is involved it is desirable to protect the fellow eye from possible contamination by using a transparent shield through which the eye may be observed (Buller's shield). Nursing attendants are advised to wear protective goggles to prevent accidental contamination.

Therapy

A conjunctival culture should be taken to determine the causal organism and its sensitivity. Then local penicillin or sulphonamide drops may be applied every five minutes for one hour before reducing the applications to hourly. In addition, supplementary therapy in the form of systemic antibiotics should appreciably minimise complications. When corneal ulceration results, guttae atropine 1% should also be applied.

Ophthalmia neonatorum is the name given to 'a purulent discharge from the eyes of an infant commencing within twenty-one days from the date of birth'. The gonococcus is commonly the causal organism but it may also result from others—staphylococcus, pneumococcus, Koch-Weeks bacillus, virus of inclusion conjunctivitis, etc.

Mucopurulent Conjunctivitis

Discharge, injection, chemosis and photophobia are noteworthy in this inflammation which may be due to the pneumococcus, staphylococcus, or the Koch-Weeks bacillus.

Pneumococcal infection usually follows obstruction in the naso-lacrimal duct and dacryocystitis, while the Koch-Weeks bacillus is often epidemic in its incidence.

A mild catarrhal or mucopurulent conjunctivitis may result from invasion by the Morax-Axenfeld diplobacillus. This infection is often restricted to the angles of the eye (i.e. around the medial and lateral canthi) where the injection and irritation are predominant.

The staphylococcus characteristically produces an acute conjunctivitis which can also be associated with a secondary marginal keratitis.

TREATMENT

It is desirable to take a conjunctival culture to determine the organisms present and their sensitivity before instituting antibiotic therapy in the form of local drops (systemic antibiotics are generally reserved for more severe infections and their complications). In acute infections, antibiotic drops should be initially applied at frequent intervals before the instillations are gradually reduced. For example, one might commence with the appropriate antibiotic drops every five minutes for half an hour, then reduce them to hourly or two hourly applications. As the condition resolves, the drops may be used three or four hourly, and then three or four times a day. Marginal keratitis necessitates the use of a mydriatic e.g. 1% atropine drops, while dark glasses will relieve photophobia.

Discharge on the lid margins is removed using cotton-wool moistened in warm water, while irrigation of conjunctiva will help to remove accumulated and infected necrotic debris and discharge.

Membranous Conjunctivitis

This form is very uncommon. An exudative membrane forms on the conjunctival surface and this membrane may be easily detached. This conjunctivitis may be due to infection by various organisms e.g. corynebacterium diphtheriae, streptococcus, gonococcus—the most characteristic form of infection is found with the diphtheria bacillus.

The disease is usually found in children suffering from or in contact with diphtheria. The lids are swollen and red while the eye is also markedly injected with the necrotic membrane on or adherent to the conjunctiva. Attempts to detach the membrane may result in haemorrhage and even subsequent scar formation.

Treatment is as for diphtheria when its causal organism is present but when one of the others is isolated recovery usually follows administration of the appropriate antibiotic.

Viral Conjunctivitis

Only two forms of conjunctivitis caused by a virus will be referred to here while its occurrence in lymphogranuloma venereum, Reiter's disease, molluscum contagiosum, vaccinia and variola may be read about elsewhere. Although follicle formation is common in viral conjunctivitis its appearance must not be interpreted as diagnostic of the condition for it also presents, for example, in allergic conjunctivitis.

Inclusion Conjunctivitis

This infection caused by one of the tric viruses is usually self-limiting and presents after a short incubation period of three or four days. There is diffuse hyperaemia and chemosis in addition to follicle formation in the tarsal conjunctiva, particularly of the lower lid. The causal virus, of venereal origin, may infect the newborn besides adults but the features in each are similar.

Trachoma

This viral infection is endemic in the Middle East and certain other parts of the world but rarely occurs in Britain, although with immigrants the active disease is occasionally seen.

After a short incubation period of about seven days a marked bilateral redness of the conjunctiva appears together with itching, a burning sensation, photophobia and lacrimation. The tarsal conjunctiva is also thickened and follicles characteristically project from the conjunctiva of the upper lid but they may be found elsewhere on the conjunctiva.

Trachoma follicles become more prominent as the disease continues, and loops of vessels grow into the cornea from the limbus (pannus), passing superficially towards the centre of the cornea. Additional lesions in the superficial cornea also occur and they take the form of epithelial erosions and keratitis which are predominant in the upper cornea.

These features may still be present when cicatrisation appears. This stage of cicatrisation incurs the disappearance of the follicles and the onset of scar tissue formation, which results in contraction and distortion of the tissues of the eyelids. The irregular white bands of scar (fibrous) tissue are subepithelial and particularly noticeable on the upper lid, but the fornices may even be partially obliterated while limbal opacification presents in the upper cornea. Later, contracture of this fibrous tissue also results in distortion of the tissues with the onset of entropion or ectropion, trichiasis, symblepharon and xerosis. The small corneal scars which are produced may be sufficiently numerous to cause impairment of vision.

Treatment of trachoma includes not only local sulphonamide or tetracycline therapy but also their systemic administration. Surgery may also be required to correct the lid deformities and corneal opacification.

Allergic Conjunctivitis

Vernal Catarrh (Spring Catarrh)

This allergic chronic disease of the conjunctiva tends to recur during warm weather in children and young people. There is intense itching, lacrimation and photophobia, while the upper palpebral conjunctiva presents an irregular cobblestone appearance. This consists of irregular flattened papillae separated from each other by fine furrows. The congested conjunctiva has a milky translucence and some mucoid discharge is also present.

Occasionally, a vernal keratitis occurs as an extension into the marginal areas of the cornea from a limbal lesion of the conjunctiva. Sometimes there is even vascularised pannus.

Treatment consists of the local application of soluble local steroids e.g. prednisolone, but in some patients it is necessary to supplement this by oral steroids. Should the follicular excrescences be prominent it may be necessary to excise them to minimise their rubbing on the cornea and line the bare area on the eyelid with a buccal mucosal graft. Guttae atropine 1% plus antibiotic drops are required for corneal involvement. In more obstinate cases, local radiotherapy may be beneficial.

Phlyctenular Keratoconjunctivitis

This is the name given to an allergic condition of the conjunctiva which often spreads to the adjacent cornea and which is probably of endogenous origin.

The lesion is initially situated in the conjunctiva adjacent to the limbus, but it can be situated anywhere in the conjunctiva. The conjunctival focus (phlycten) ulcerates in its centre, presenting a yellow coloration which is surrounded by a red hyperaemic cuff which itself may spread to give a more widespread conjunctival injection. Spontaneous cure without cicatrisation is the rule in untreated cases after a few days, although the whole condition only lasts for a few weeks.

Treatment consists of local steroid drops, but in secondary infection antibiotic drops are also utilised.

Allergic conjunctivitis also arises from contact with substances to which the particular individual is sensitive. In ophthalmic practice, this is sometimes seen with therapeutic application of atropine, eserine and some antibiotics. The skin of the lids becomes swollen, eczematous and there is intense conjunctival hyperaemia besides epiphora.

Treatment consists of cessation or withdrawal of the causal irritant. In addition, administration of anti-allergic drugs, e.g. Otrivine-Antistin or steroids affords considerable relief.

TRAUMA

Foreign bodies may enter the conjunctival sac and give rise to local irritation or redness of the conjunctiva. Removal of the foreign body is generally easy. Occasionally, a foreign body may be impacted in the conjunctiva of the upper lid and, here, the removal is effected after eversion of the lid.

Large foreign bodies can lacerate the conjunctiva, but when the tear is small surgical repair is unnecessary. On the other hand, large lacerations should be sutured with silk or 6/0 catgut.

Laceration of the conjunctiva frequently causes rupture of one of the conjunctival vessels and subconjunctival haemorrhage. Although the bright red haemorrhage may be large it absorbs without complication during the ensuing days or weeks.

Chemical burns arise when chemical irritants e.g. acids or alkalis enter the eyelids. The irritant causes redness of the conjunctiva which is often more marked in the lower fornix. Ideally, the irritant should be immediately washed out by copious lavage with the eyelids widely opened. Lavage, in the first instance, may have to be restricted to water or saline.

Lime burns are often seen and, because of the possibility of lime particles being retained in the conjunctiva, they deserve assiduous attention. The lime causes tissue necrosis which is followed by cicatrisation, and opacification of the cornea is also seen.

Fibrous tissue cicatrisation gives rise to bands which stretch between the eyeball and the eyelid, thereby obliterating the conjunctival fornix.

The conjunctival fornices should be freely and immediately irrigated, preferably after the instillation of anaesthetic drops (to overcome the blepharospasm). Di-sodium versonate (1% solution) is probably most beneficial if it is available otherwise saline or water will suffice for lavage. A camel hair brush and liquid paraffin facilitates removal of impacted lime particles. Adhesions between the globe and eyelids may be prevented by daily passing a glass rod around the fornices till healing is complete. The glass rod may be used in conjunction with oculentum cortisone (the steroid minimises the fibrosis) but, when the damaged area is extensive, the temporary fitting of a contact lens is often desirable. Severe damage to the conjunctiva generally requires surgical repair.

Implantation Cyst

Sometimes following injury, fragments of conjunctiva may become impacted subconjunctivally. These cysts slowly enlarge and, therefore, early excision is indicated.

CONJUNCTIVITIS AND DISORDERS OF THE SKIN

This association perhaps occurs more frequently than is suspected, for many of the milder disorders pass unnoticed.

Acne Rosacea

Acne rosacea is one disorder in which cutaneous changes occur over the cheeks and nose while there is also a well-marked blepharo-conjunctivitis. Often there is an additional keratitis (rosacea keratitis) which is characterised by superficial infiltrates in the lower cornea, sometimes with tongue or horse-shoe shaped opacities into which leashes of superficial vessels grow from the limbus. Although response to steroid therapy is good, recurrence is the rule.

Pemphigus

Pemphigus may occur as part of a generalised pemphigus or present as an entirely localised entity. When the eye is involved, the disease starts in the conjunctiva but there is early subconjunctival fibrosis which undergoes contracture. These develop into symblepharon and give inadequate lid closure with its resultant exposure keratitis in addition to keratinisation. Treatment is a problem in some, but steroid therapy does afford relief.

Erythema Multiforme (Stevens-Johnson Syndrome)

This is characterised by widespread exudative lesions of the hands, arms and neck, and of the conjunctiva, nose, mouth and genital passages. Sepsis in the lesions may present a sinister appearance but most patients recover spontaneously although there is a tendency to treat them with systemic antibiotics, sometimes in conjunction with steroids.

DEGENERATIONS

Pinguecula

This takes the form of a yellowish, slightly raised nodule situated on the interpalpebral conjunctiva on either side of the cornea. Histologically, it consists of a hyaline degeneration and its excision is rarely required.

Pterygium

This degenerative condition generally starts as a tongue-shaped vascular mass on the nasal side of the cornea. Encroachment on the cornea is the rule but this varies in its extent. Again, there is hyaline degeneration and subepithelial fibrosis. Surgery is indicated if extension onto the cornea progresses but the multitudinous manoeuvres only indicate how unsatisfactory many are.

Cystic degeneration or change may take place in the conjunctiva. These thin-walled translucent cysts may be removed by simple excision.

TUMOURS

Benign Tumours

Papilloma

This benign epithelioma may be located anywhere on the conjunctiva. Its vascular core frequently draws attention to its presence. Treatment consists of excision.

Simple Melanoma (Naevus)

This neoplasm frequently pigments around puberty and thereby becomes more easily noticed. It is commonly situated near the limbus. Although benign, excision may be desirable for cosmetic reasons but is also indicated when there is an increase in size.

Malignant Tumours

Epithelioma

This may arise anywhere in the conjunctiva where it appears as an irregular vascularised mass which is locally invasive and which may metastasise to the regional lymph nodes. Adequate excision is the most satisfactory line of treatment.

Rodent Ulcer (basal cell carcinoma)

Most commonly situated near the inner canthus, this neoplasm tends to ulcerate in its centre which has a raised, reddish surround to the ulcer. Treatment is by excision or by radiotherapy (which must be expertly administered).

Malignant Melanoma

Rarely it commences in a naevus when the tumour forms a raised irregular pigmented mass which gradually spreads with a tendency to ulcerate and to evoke a surrounding reactionary hyperaemia. Treatment depends on the extent of spread, which may necessitate only simple excision or even involve as much as exenteration, if extensive.

4 *DISEASES OF THE CORNEA*

ANATOMY

The cornea is the transparent anterior one-sixth of the external coat of the eyeball. The average diameter of the cornea is about 11 mm. The cornea is composed of the following layers (from its anterior or superficial surface to the deep one):

(1) Epithelium. A stratified non-keratinised structure which is continuous at the periphery of the cornea (limbus) with the conjunctiva.

(2) Bowman's membrane. A thin homogeneous membrane, which is closely connected with the stroma.

(3) Stroma. This layer constituting the bulk of the cornea, consists of lamellae of collagen fibrils which are largely parallel. Lying in the stroma are branching cells (corneal corpuscles and nerve fibrils). At the periphery of the cornea, the stroma is continuous with the sclera.

(4) Endothelium. This is a single layer of hexagonal cells which is in contact with the aqueous humour. The integrity of the endothelium is an important factor in the maintenance of corneal transparency.

Damage to the corneal epithelium or its absence may be demonstrated by the use of fluorescein. A drop of a 2% solution of fluorescein is instilled, and any defective areas of epithelium take on a bright green coloration (the excess precorneal fluorescein is removed by saline lavage). Another dye which may be similarly used is Bengal Rose (1%) but here the coloration is red.

CONGENITAL ABNORMALITIES

Microcornea

A small cornea may occur in an otherwise normal eye but, in others, the eye as a whole may be small (microphthalmos). Refraction generally reveals hypermetropia, and maldevelopment involving the filtration angle predisposes to glaucoma.

Megalocornea

There is obvious enlargement of the cornea but this may also be associated with other changes in the anterior segment of the eye which itself is myopic.

INFLAMMATION

Keratitis

Keratitis is the name given to inflammations of the cornea which may be either endogenous or exogenous (bacterial, viral or mycotic). By far the more common is the exogenous form. Healthy cornea is transparent and avascular but in keratitis, there are infiltration and necrosis which result in opacification and even vascular invasion from the nearest part of the limbus. These ingrowing vessels may be superficial or deep. Occasionally, extensive destruction of the cornea results in its perforation and thus provides a ready track for infection to enter the eye.

Bacterial Keratitis

A wide variety of organisms may cause this: *Staphylococcus, Streptococcus, Pneumococcus, Pseudomonas pyocyanea, Gonococcus, B. proteus* and *B. coli*. The eye is painful, and there are blepharospasm, lacrimation and photophobia while circumcorneal (ciliary) injection is the rule. When ulceration has destroyed the epithelium, fluorescein 1% solution will demonstrate the extent of the destruction (corneal ulcer). There is greyish-white coloration of the infiltrated area of cornea and corneal excavation in more severe ulcers while oedema may involve the adjacent cornea. A reflex iritis is common with most forms of keratitis. An ulcer may be peripheral when the spread is from an adjacent conjunctival infection or in others (especially pneumococcus) the ulcer is more central. Milder infections tend to heal without neovascularisation and with only slight opacification (nebula) but in more severe ones the opacity is dense (leucoma). An ulcer causes marked stromal destruction, and then the unsupported Descemet's membrane protrudes externally (Descemetocoele). Perforation of the cornea occurs if the highly resistant Descemet's membrane is breached—aqueous is then expressed through the rupture. Escape of aqueous results in a forward movement of the iris which may then become impacted in the perforation or even protrude through it (iris prolapse). Adhesion of the iris to the damaged cornea (anterior synechia) may become permanent while the diseased or damaged cornea may protrude forwards (anterior staphyloma). During active ulceration, pus may gather in the anterior chamber (hypopyon) and spread of infection within the eye (panophthalmitis) results in extensive destruction with subsequent shrinkage (phthisis bulbi).

Treatment

Early and frequent local applications of antibiotics are essential but, before commencing this, it is desirable to take a culture to determine the sensitivity of any organisms present. In severe ulceration, a more effective concentration of antibiotic is obtained by subconjunctival injection of selected antibiotics. A mydriatic is essential to overcome the iritis and atropine 1% (guttae or oculentum) is usually employed. The eye is more comfortable if kept closed by an eye-pad, and further relief results from heat applied to the eye by hot spoon bathing or electric eye pad.

Carbolisation or cauterization of the ulcer was formerly common but is rare nowadays. Indolent ulceration frequently responds to tarsorrhaphy.

VIRAL KERATITIS

Herpes Simplex

This is the term utilised for a viral involvement of the corneal epithelium which is characterised by numerous vesicular foci staining with Bengal Rose. These are usually associated with whitish subepithelial lesions. A not uncommon precursor is a herpetic vesicular eruption on the face or respiratory infection e.g. common cold.

Herpetic Keratitis

This keratitis forms a distinctive branching line of epithelial vesiculation which quickly breaks down to form a continuous ulcer resembling the branches of a tree in outline. It often follows an upper respiratory infection. Although initially an epithelial infection, it is liable to spread to the stroma where the infection gives a stromal infiltration with haziness of the cornea and impairment of vision. Because of its rounded shape, this stromal involvement is referred to as disciform keratitis. Unfortunately, the stromal opacification may persist and even become infiltrated by ingrowing blood vessels which grow deeply into the cornea from the limbal plexus.

Many dendritic ulcers tend to gradually spread so that extensive areas of ulceration result. These ulcers show an *increased* tendency to extend rapidly if cortisone is given. Once resolution of the ulcer takes place, recurrence may subsequently occur at any time.

Treatment

It is essential to start treatment early and to obtain resolution in order to minimise corneal scarring; ideally, therefore, at the onset of epithelial involvement. Many dendritic ulcers heal well when guttae I.D.U. (5 iodo-2-deoxyuridine) are used hourly; this intensive therapy is essential. Alternatively, the ulcer may be cauterised with iodine or phenol but this must be done carefully to avoid unnecessary corneal destruction. Indolent dendritic ulceration may sometimes require tarsorrhaphy (union of the eyelids) while sometimes the diseased segment of cornea is removed and healthy cornea from a donor eye is grafted into the area (corneal graft or keratoplasty).

Disciform Keratitis

The use of local steroids is advocated in disciform keratitis when no active epithelial lesions are present.

Epidemic Kerato-conjunctivitis

An adenovirus is the causal organism in this infection consisting of localised subepithelial infiltrations. These hazy lesions are usually transient and heal without any scarring. The ocular infection is accompanied by enlargement of the preauricular lymph nodes.

Herpes Zoster Ophthalmicus

This usually follows a previous chicken-pox infection and suggests that a common virus is responsible for both. In herpes zoster ophthalmicus, the virus affects the trigeminal ganglion or the ophthalmic division of the trigeminal nerve.

The onset is dramatic and sudden with marked neuralgic pain along the distribution of the trigeminal nerve on one side (between the tip of the nose and the occiput). After a few hours, redness and vesiculation appears along the distribution of the nerve. The conjunctiva becomes injected and some mucopurulent discharge may be present but corneal involvement commences with vesiculation and stromal opacification. Initially, the corneal staining with fluorescein is small but the staining foci may coalesce to give a large one which leaves opacification. It is important to watch for keratic precipitates (K.P.) on the corneal endothelium—these herald uveal involvement and may lead to secondary glaucoma. In some cases, the corneal nerves may be extensively damaged and the cornea is anaesthetic, a condition known as neurotrophic keratitis.

Treatment is largely symptomatic. An antibiotic and steroid oculentum may be applied to the eye while atropine counteracts the uveitis. If secondary glaucoma supervenes, this treatment may be supplemented with tab. Diamox (acetazolamide) 250 mg once to thrice daily. Corneal anaesthesia may require tarsorrhaphy.

Mycotic Keratitis

This infection is uncommon and characterised by a relapsing keratitis with periods of remission. A yellowish infiltration is present in the involved area which has a hazy surrounding halo. Rarely does the fungal infection give rise to a hypopyon. Treatment consists of the administration of anti-fungal agents e.g. Amphotericin.

Interstitial Keratitis

The majority of patients with this condition have congenital syphilis but others may suffer from tuberculosis, one of the tropical diseases or lupus erythematosus, and it may appear as a sequel to a viral infection of the cornea or a severe anterior uveitis.

Initially, central cloudiness of the cornea spreads to involve most of it while the cornea becomes progressively more opacified. The visual acuity is grossly reduced in an eye which is not only red but intensely painful. An intense iritis also develops while blepharospasm and photophobia add to the discomfort. Blood vessels grow into the deeper stroma giving the cornea a salmon pink hue. The marked corneal inflammation gives a severe opacification which is permanent. As resolution progresses, the outlines of empty blood vessels (ghost vessels) in the cornea are evident and the patient may obtain remarkably good vision although, on the other hand, it may be greatly reduced. Evidence of uveitis is also present. Interstitial keratitis is characteristically bilateral.

Treatment

Steroids greatly reduce corneal damage while atropine is essential for the uveitis; where syphilis is the causal factor an active treatment for it is essential. When extensive corneal opacification is present, keratoplasty often gives good results.

Neuroparalytic Keratitis

This condition may follow facial paresis or exophthalmos when the cornea is exposed. The lack of protection normally afforded by the eyelids leads to dehydration and desquamation of the cornea. Infection of the damaged cornea may quickly appear and even proceed to abscess formation in the cornea.

TREATMENT

Tarsorrhaphy is effective in protecting the cornea, but abscess formation also requires local and systemic antibiotics.

DEGENERATIONS

Arcus Senilis

This consists of a white band concentric with the limbus from which it is separated by a narrow area of clear cornea. Histologically, it is a lipoid degeneration of the stroma adjacent to Bowman's membrane. No treatment is required as the condition is symptom free.

Band Degeneration

This may be idiopathic when it occurs in a previously healthy cornea but is usually secondary to chronic inflammation or to glaucoma. It consists of a fine greyish-white band which stretches across the cornea normally exposed when the lids are open. There is a hyaline and calcareous degeneration in the region of Bowman's membrane.

TREATMENT

The degenerate area may be removed with the aid of disodium versonate drops after much of the degenerate cornea has been scraped away but sometimes keratoplasty may be needed to replace opacified cornea by clear cornea.

Mustard Gas Keratitis

This condition is largely confined to soldiers exposed to this toxic gas during the 1914–18 war. Mild exposure causes immediate conjunctival irritation but in severe exposure the necrotising gas gives corneal ulceration and opacification. Eventually the ulcer heals but it may leave a dense scar which reduces vision. The conjunctival vessels are also involved and form aneurysmal dilatations near the limbus besides invading the diseased cornea. Treatment is largely symptomatic but contact lenses may be of use and keratoplasty is advocated in some.

Keratoconjunctivitis Sicca

Deficient secretion of tears produces focal corneal and conjunctival desiccation which stains vividly with Bengal Rose. The eyes are photophobic and irritable, and secondary infecton may give corneal ulceration. A white stringy discharge from the conjunctiva is common. Once established, the condition tends to persist. The deficiency of tears is usually accompanied by a similar lack of saliva and by arthritis (Sjogren's syndrome).

TREATMENT

Relief may be given to patients by the repeated instillation of artificial tears but alkaline methyl cellulose 1% is more effective as it remains in contact with the eye for longer. Cauterisation of the lacrimal puncta prevents the drainage of tears thereby retaining them to moisten the eye. Oculentum chloramphenicol is often useful in combating secondary infection.

Mooren's Ulcer

This chronic, slowly progressive, often painful ulcer begins near the upper margin of the cornea into which it slowly advances with an overhanging edge. Initially, it is unilateral, and the ulcer produces a deep destruction of the cornea as it gradually spreads to involve much of the cornea. The thinned remnants of cornea are opacified and vascularised besides being ectatic in some. Treatment is generally of no avail but in some cases steroids have been of limited value.

CORNEAL DYSTROPHIES

Endothelial and Epithelial Dystrophy (Fuchs')

This bilateral dystrophy commences in the endothelium which presents an irregular mottled appearance with scattered bronzed or refractile particles and dark vacuolated areas. It generally appears after forty years of age. The damaged endothelium is permeable to aqueous and the oedematous stroma becomes hazy while, later, oedematous bullae in the epithelium may rupture and cause pain. Finally, the entire cornea becomes opaque. The process tends to be accelerated by intraocular surgery e.g. cataract extraction.

Nodular Dystrophy (Groenouw's)

Opacities appear in the stroma in the central region, often about the age of puberty.

Keratoconus

This form of corneal dystrophy usually becomes evident around puberty, when the cornea protrudes forward and becomes ectatic. This tends to progress slowly and myopic astigmatism develops. Ruptures appear in Descemet's membrane together with opacities in the stroma which may have an annular form.

Treatment

It is worth while trying patients who have a corneal dystrophy with contact lenses but most do well with keratoplasty. If the dystrophy is superficial, a lamellar graft will suffice but for deeper corneal involvement a penetrating keratoplasty is needed.

PIGMENTATION OF THE CORNEA

Melanin

A fine brown horizontal line may appear in the lower cornea after about fifty years of age (Hudson-Stahli line). An elongated aggregation of pigment granules can gather on the endothelium (Krukenberg's spindle).

Haematogenous Pigmentation

Blood-staining of the cornea occurs in some cases of hyphaema when blood permeates into the cornea which assumes a brownish coloration. Penetration of the cornea is promoted by raised intraocular tension and in patients with a damaged endothelium e.g. endothelial dystrophy. Blood-staining may also follow intra-corneal or subconjunctival haemorrhage.

Kayser-Fleischer ring is a green-brown ring situated in the peripheral cornea, superficial to Descemet's membrane. The ring is an early manifestation of hepato-lenticular degeneration and is believed to be derived from haematogenous pigment, although some workers have found copper in it.

Exogenous Pigmentation

Small particles of iron, copper or silver may be deposited in the cornea. The latter deposition (argyrosis) occurs most frequently after an excessive intake of silver while the former (siderosis and chalcosis respectively) are generally associated with retained foreign bodies.

Antimalarial Drugs

Chloroquine, in particular, when administered in excess, is liable to give rise to the deposition of whitish granules in the superficial stroma. These granules gather in characteristic whorls in the cornea, which may or may not be accompanied by a pigmentary degeneration of the retina.

Corneal neoplasms are particularly rare but endotheliomata and melanomata are amongst the more common of them.

5 *DISEASES OF THE SCLERA*

ANATOMY

The sclera forms the posterior five sixths of the outer coat of the eyeball. It is whitish in colour, about 1 mm thick, being largely composed of connective tissue. The sclera is pierced about 2·5 mm medial to the posterior pole of the eye by the optic nerve and elsewhere by smaller nerves and by blood vessels. The extrinsic ocular muscles gain attachment to the sclera.

Inflammation of the Sclera

Episcleritis is an inflammation of the superficial sclera, but inflammation may involve the sclera generally when it is referred to as scleritis.

Episcleritis

This is usually a localised superficial inflammation which has a characteristic dusky-red colour and there is some oedema of the episclera which is also tender on palpation. Unlike conjunctivitis, there is no lacrimation, no discharge and no photophobia. Resolution is generally quick but may be delayed for some weeks. Relapses are not uncommon. Episcleritis is included amongst the collagen diseases and tends to respond well to steroids.

Scleritis

The entire thickness of sclera is affected and sometimes the inflammation may spread to involve the adjacent cornea (sclerosing keratitis). In others, uveitis may accompany the scleritis. The clinical features are much the same as in episcleritis, but the sclera may become thinned and assume a blue colour besides being ectatic (staphyloma). Treatment is with steroids or A.C.T.H.

6 *DISEASES OF THE UVEAL TRACT*

ANATOMY

The uvea is the vascular or middle coat of the eyeball and traditionally is described as consisting, from before backwards, of iris, ciliary body and choroid which are continuous.

The iris is a circular coloured membrane which forms part of the posterior limits of the anterior chamber. The posterior surface of the iris helps to constitute part of the boundary of the posterior chamber. Thus, the anterior and posterior surfaces of the iris are bathed by aqueous humour which also flows through the opening near the centre of the iris (pupil). The average size of the pupil is 4 mm. The pupil is in constant movement (hippus) undergoing dilatation (due to the dilatator pupillae muscle of the iris) and constriction (sphincter pupillae muscle).

The anterior surface of the iris is covered by a single layer of epithelium while deep to it is the bulk of the iris—the stroma. It consists of a delicate connective tissue with radially running blood vessels together with stromal pigment which gives the colour to the iris. The sphincter pupillae surrounds the pupil in the thinner part of the iris which itself merges with the thicker part at a junction known as the collarette. In the thicker part of the iris is the radially placed fibrils of the dilatator pupillae muscle. Posterior to these muscle fibres are the two layers of epithelium, (1) the pigmented layer is continuous with the pigment epithelium of the ciliary body, (2) the non-pigmented epithelium likewise continuous with a similar epithelium of the ciliary body.

The sphincter pupillae is supplied by the third cranial nerve and the dilatator pupillae by the sympathetic nervous system.

The *ciliary body* is that portion of the uvea between the root of the iris and the anterior part of the choroid. The ciliary muscle of somewhat triangular outline forms the bulk of the ciliary body, and lies towards its outer part. This muscle is non-striated while its contraction causes forward and inward movement of the ciliary processes and relaxation of the suspensory ligament of the lens which itself becomes more convex. The fibro-vascular tissue of the iris and choroid is continuous with that around the ciliary muscle. The innermost part of the ciliary body is divided into two segments, the posterior smooth portion called the pars plana and an irregularly ridged anterior one with the ciliary processes. These are lined by two layers of epithelium, pigmented and non-pigmented. There are about seventy meridionally placed folds with vascular cores known as ciliary processes. The epithelium of the processes is concerned with the secretion of aqueous humour and the processes have a rich vascular supply, (1) the arterial system arises from the greater arterial circle of the iris and the anterior ciliary arteries, (2) the veins drain posteriorly to the venae vorticosae of the choroid but some anteriorly placed veins emerge from the sclera in company with the anterior ciliary arteries.

The ciliary muscle is innervated by the oculomotor nerve (third cranial). The stimulus for accommodation arises in the occipital cortex and passes via the parasympathetic part of the oculomotor nucleus to the ciliary ganglion, where it is relayed to the ciliary muscle which contracts.

The choroid is the dark brown vascular tissue stretching from the ora serrata to the optic nerve and lying between the retina and sclera. The large vessels of the choroid are situated superficially and the vessels gradually decrease in size towards the interior of

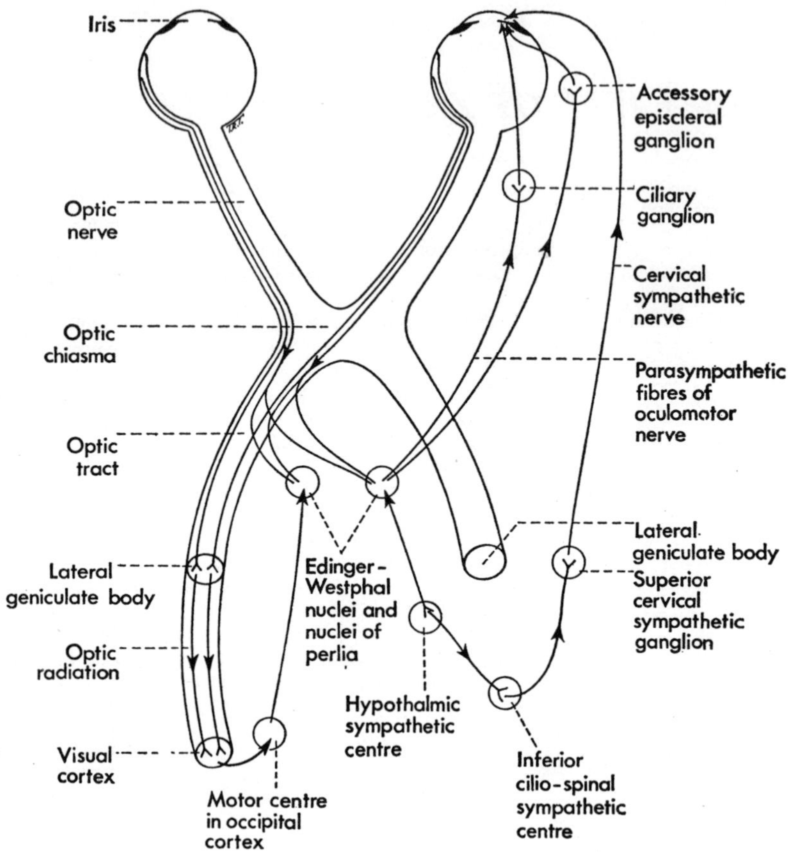

FIG 13 Nerve pathways of the pupillary light and accommodation reflexes (*after Wybar*)

the choroid where the fine capillaries are called the choriocapillaris. Amidst the blood vessels, are the pigment cells of somewhat stellate outline, and which are responsible for the dark brown colour of the choroid. Nutrition to the outer retina passes from these vessels through the structureless homogeneous membrane of Bruch (which is the innermost part of the choroid).

CONGENITAL ABNORMALITIES

Persistent Pupillary Membrane

A delicate vascular mesodermal membrane closes the pupillary area in the foetus within the collarette. Normally, this membrane absorbs before birth, but sometimes the absorption is incomplete and strands remain in the anterior chamber where they may remain attached to the iris, or run between the iris and anterior lens capsule or lie freely in the anterior chamber. Rudimentary elements of the membrane are sometimes present on the anterior lens capsule as brown stellate deposits (epicapsular stars).

Aniridia

In this condition, only rudimentary elements of the iris exist in the region of the filtration angle where they are largely hidden behind the corneo-scleral margin. The absence of large areas of iris allows light to pass unimpeded and causes photophobia. Congenital nystagmus is usually present as are glaucoma and lens opacities in early life. Relief from photophobia may be obtained with tinted spectacle lenses or contact lenses.

Coloboma of the Iris and Choroid

Failure of closure of the foetal cleft leaves a defect in the uvea which is usually situated below and nasally. This defect may only involve a small segment of iris or the defect may even extend as far as the lower border of the optic disc. This condition is usually bilateral but seldom of equal extent in both eyes. Coloboma of the iris gives a characteristic 'keyhole' appearance to the pupil while a coloboma of the choroid exposes the white sclera.

Albinism

This hereditary condition is characterised not only by a deficiency of uveal pigment but also in the whole body. This gives a pink colour to the eye which is photophobic and myopic. The poor macular fixation also present results in nystagmus. Dark glasses and contact lenses are often beneficial.

INFLAMMATION

Inflammation of the uveal tract is referred to as uveitis. It may involve the entire uvea (pan-uveitis or endophthalmitis), or only part of the uvea e.g. anterior uvea (anterior uveitis). When the inflammation is largely resident in the iris, it is often referred to as iritis, while inflammation of the ciliary body is sometimes known as cyclitis or iridocyclitis. A posterior uveitis or choroiditis is inflammation of the choroid.

Anterior Uveitis (Iritis or Iridocyclitis) (Plates 4 and 5)

The onset consists of an ache or pain in or around the eye with photophobia and impaired vision of a variable amount.

Clinical examination reveals lacrimation and circumcorneal injection (ciliary injection). The most important sign in the tender eyeball is the presence of inflammatory cells in the anterior chamber which may even be hazy (aqueous flare). These cells and a hazy exudate pass from the inflamed uvea into the aqueous (which also circulates immediately behind the lens in the retrolental space). Some of the inflammatory cells may be deposited on the corneal endothelium where they are referred to as keratic precipitates (K.P.). The K.P. usually form a triangular outline on the endothelium but sometimes they are widely disseminated over the corneal endothelium e.g. heterochromic cyclitis. K.P. vary in number and size: large, non-pigmented K.P. (mutton-fat K.P.) are suggestive of tuberculosis and sarcoidosis, and crenated pigmented K.P. are indicative of a chronic inflammation.

When the inflammatory exudate is excessive it accumulates in the lower part of the anterior chamber (hypopyon). The iris assumes a greenish muddy colour, becomes oedematous and its engorged vessels are prominent. They are liable to bleed, giving rise to a hyphaema. The oedematous iris readily adheres to the adjacent anterior surface of the lens (posterior synechiae). The pupil becomes constricted, only dilating with difficulty. Dilation of the pupil may sever some of these synechiae and this leaves irregular clumps of iris pigment on the anterior surface of the lens, but in others the synechiae persist and allow only irregular dilatation of the pupil.

The toxicity may be marked enough to involve the cornea which then also becomes hazy and oedematous. The intraocular tension is usually normal but when the exudation gathers in or obstructs the filtration spaces the tension rises. Another cause of raised tension is the formation of a ring of posterior synechiae around the pupillary margin (seclusio pupillae), thus preventing the forward flow of aqueous from the posterior chamber through the pupil into the anterior chamber. Thus, the pressure of aqueous builds up behind the iris which becomes bowed forwards (iris bombé).

Persistence of the corneal oedema may in time leave opacification of the cornea, while the toxic aqueous leads to defective nourishment of the lens and the onset of lenticular opacities (cataract). Repeated or protracted inflammation may ultimately lead to atrophy of the uvea (atrophia bulbi).

Posterior Uveitis (Choroiditis)

Visual disturbances in the nature of 'spots in front of the eye', distortion of objects or blurred vision herald the onset of this inflammation. The vitreous becomes hazy due to the accumulation in it of inflammatory cells which have migrated into the vitreous from the inflamed uvea. Because of the intimate contact with the retina, inflammation in the choroid usually involves the retina (choroido-retinitis).

In the acute stage, the inflammatory focus of choroiditis presents a fuzzy or indistinct white swelling over which the retinal vessels may be seen to course. The patch or patches may be situated in any part of the choroid and be of varying shape and size.

The damaged retina produces a defect in the visual field (scotoma) which initially corresponds in shape with the retinal lesion. On the other hand, extension of the inflammation to involve the nerve fibrils gives a sector-shaped field defect. In some patients, the uveitis may become chronic and persist but most resolve satisfactorily.

When the choroiditis impairs macular function, central vision is diminished, but choroiditis adjacent to the optic disc (juxtapapillary choroiditis) tends to give a sectorial field defect because of involvement of nerve fibrils. Peripheral choroiditis may even pass undetected.

Pan Uveitis

Widespread oedema of the retina is common as a result of this infection but it must be remembered that an anterior uveitis is also present. The inflammation may involve the optic disc which is initially oedematous but later atrophic. Resolution reveals choroido-retinal atrophy with poor vision.

Treatment

Milder forms of anterior uveitis may be adequately treated using sufficient mydriatic to dilate the pupil, e.g. guttae atropine 1% or 2%, guttae hyoscine ¼% or ½% are probably most commonly used perhaps because of their long duration of action. This may, however, be supplemented by guttae phenylephrine 10% or guttae cyclopentolate 1% (mydrilate); the action of both is shorter. In addition, local steroids are beneficial and here guttae or oculentum is often adequate. The anterior uveitis may be more severe and the above regime may not suffice so that subconjunctival injections of steroids may be required in addition to a subconjunctival injection of mydricaine.

Local steroids are insufficient in choroiditis and one must revert to oral steroids. A search must be made for the causal factor and its treatment instituted.

Sympathetic Ophthalmitis

This is the term utilised for a plastic inflammation of the uvea in one eye (sympathising eye) following a perforating injury in the fellow eye (exciting eye). Trauma to the uvea of the exciting eye is usual and this is followed by a latent period of at least ten days following the injury. In some, the latent period may extend to months or even years before the onset of photophobia and lacrimation in the sympathising eye. The vision becomes blurred while cells and a flare appear in the aqueous before the deposition of keratic precipitates. The margins of the optic disc may be blurred and as the inflammation continues posterior synechiae occur. In the late stages, vitreous opacities, secondary cataract and exudative separation of the retina appear. The terminal result in untreated cases is phthisis bulbi.

Treatment

The injured eye should be enucleated if it is blind but if good vision is a likelihood then the exciting eye should be retained. If enucleation is chosen, it should be early and before the onset of inflammation in the uninjured eye as enucleation of the injured eye after sympathetic ophthalmitis is established does not necessarily arrest the inflammation. Intensive treatment with substantial doses of oral steroids is probably the most effective therapy.

Panophthalmitis

This is a severe purulent inflammation of the entire uvea which generally follows a penetrating injury but which, more rarely, may be metastatic from a blood-borne infection. The infection is severe with pain, chemosis, intense redness of the eye and corneal oedema. Pus accumulates within the eye and may eventually fill the globe which is then blind.

The only treatment is early and adequate systemic antibiotic. However, once vision is lost, evisceration may be desirable.

Toxoplasmosis

Infestation by the causal protozoa may cause widespread infection involving the central nervous system, liver and lymphatic system besides the eye. In the eye, choroiditis in the posterior fundus typically presents heavy pigment deposition at the edges of the focus. The early toxoplasmic focus is white with fluffy edges, but as it resolves pigmentation appears. Congenital infection may result in additional lesions: nystagmus, microphthalmos and cataract. The toxoplasmosis methylene blue dye test in the blood may aid in diagnosis.

Treatment

Pyrimethamine (Daraprim) 25 mg daily or twice daily in conjunction with oral sulphonamides (one tablet three times a day), for fourteen days is of value. When the inflammation involves the macular area or the papillo-macular fibres, it is desirable to supplement the above with oral steroids in an endeavour to minimise damage to these important visual elements.

Tuberculosis

This now rarely involves the uvea probably because of its diminished incidence elsewhere in the body nowadays.

The uveitis may be anterior or posterior. In the former, large 'mutton-fat' K.P. are deposited on the cornea. Treatment is as for generalised tuberculosis.

Sarcoidosis

Large white K.P. in profusion are prominent in this condition while small white sarcoid nodules may appear on the anterior surface of the iris near its pupillary margin. Sarcoidosis is usually also demonstrable elsewhere: lymph glands (especially hilar), subcutaneous, bones, and lungs. The Mantoux reaction is negative.

Sarcoidosis may be present in (1) both the uvea and salivary glands (Heerfordt's disease or uveo-parotid fever) giving a uveitis and parotid inflammation, (2) Mikulicz's syndrome (uveitis and involvement of the lacrimal gland).

Response to oral steroids is often dramatic.

Syphilis

Congenital syphilis may give rise to an anterior uveitis while activity remains in interstitial keratitis. Rarely, a widespread pigmentary degeneration in both fundi results from congenital luetic infection. The appearances are characteristically described as 'pepper and salt'.

Anterior uveitis also occurs in acquired syphilis but a posterior uveitis is more rare.

Still's Disease

A rheumatoid arthritis, especially involving the lower limbs, is characteristic of this disease of childhood which is also associated with bilateral anterior uveitis. In some cases a posterior uveitis is also present. The uveitis tends to be chronic and secondary cataract and glaucoma are prone to occur. As the infection continues a band-shaped degeneration of the cornea also appears. Systemic steroids give the most satisfactory improvement.

Heterochromic Cyclitis

This condition commonly presents in otherwise healthy young adults. Typically, it is unilateral and runs a chronic course over years. Despite the inflammation, the eye is generally white, but white crenated K.P. are widely deposited over the whole corneal endothelium. Occasional cells are present in the anterior chamber while there is also depigmentation of the iris. No posterior synechiae are present between the iris and lens which itself becomes more opacified. Lens extraction may improve vision provided the vitreous opacities are not too numerous. Occasionally glaucoma appears. Treatment of the uveitis seems to do little to impede continuance of the cyclitis.

INJURIES

Hyphaema

Bleeding into the anterior chamber may come from the iris or ciliary body following injury to the eye. The extent of the haemorrhage varies in amount from only a slight extravasation to an extensive one filling the anterior chamber. The red blood cells may become impacted in the filtration spaces thereby blocking drainage of aqueous and causing the onset of secondary glaucoma. With this raised pressure, haematogenous pigment accumulates in the cornea giving it a brownish coloration, blood staining of the cornea. In most cases, the hyphaema absorbs satisfactorily but when the intraocular tension rises it is desirable to reduce the intraocular pressure with acetazolamide (Diamox) but, if this does not suffice, evacuation of the hyphaema by surgery is required.

Iridodialysis

Injury to the iris may result in tearing of its substance. The tear is usually at the iris root and the opening persists because union of the torn edges of the iris does not occur.

Traumatic Mydriasis or Miosis

A blunt injury to the eye may result in mydriasis due to paralysis of the sphincter pupillae. Occasionally, miosis follows injury.

Hypotonia sometimes follows trauma to the ciliary body, while a penetrating injury tears the ciliary body.

The choroid may also be damaged. Choroidal haemorrhage, red or dark blue in colour, may be large or small. Rupture of the choroid generally commences with a choroidal haemorrhage which gradually absorbs to expose a narrow whitish crescent area of atrophy. Usually concentric with the temporal border of the optic disc, the choroidal tear is crossed by the retinal vessels.

DEGENERATION OF THE UVEA

Colloid Degeneration

These bodies are situated on Bruch's membrane near the posterior pole and are believed to be ischaemic in origin. Ophthalmoscopically, colloid bodies have a yellowish appearance and characteristically do not impair vision.

Myopic Degeneration

In myopia, the choroid frequently shows a white crescentic area of atrophy along the temporal border of the optic disc (myopic crescent): in more marked cases the atrophy encircles the optic papilla.

In high myopia the sclera may bulge posteriorly, the ectasia being referred to as a posterior staphyloma.

Choroidal Sclerosis

In this condition, there is a degeneration of the choriocapillaris which selectively involves only the posterior pole making the vessels more prominent and whitish.

Disciform Degeneration

Haemorrhage in the choroid from degenerate choroidal vessels at the posterior pole is often the first manifestation of this condition which is seen more often in the aged. The first ophthalmoscopic features are white retinal exudates often arranged in an annular manner around the macula (retinitis circinata). In others, a choroidal haemorrhage presenting a dark blue swelling in the macular area is the first presentation. It is accompanied by a deterioration in vision which usually persists. The area of haemorrhage gradually absorbs but this is accompanied by retinal atrophy. Treatment is of no avail.

TUMOURS

Benign

Angioma

This cavernous tumour is most commonly seen in the choroid. Often it tends to be associated with a port-wine naevus flammeus of the ipsilateral side of the face and glaucoma. Outside the eye, angiomatous formations may be found in the cerebral cortex and meninges (Sturge-Weber syndrome).

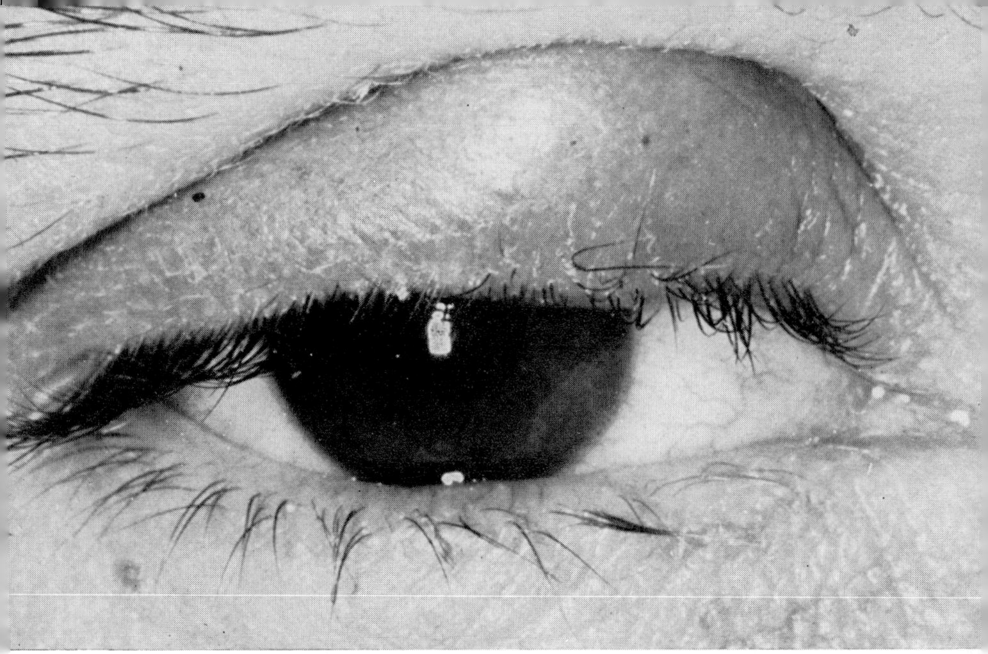

PLATE 1 Chalazion in upper lid

PLATE 2 Conjunctival injection

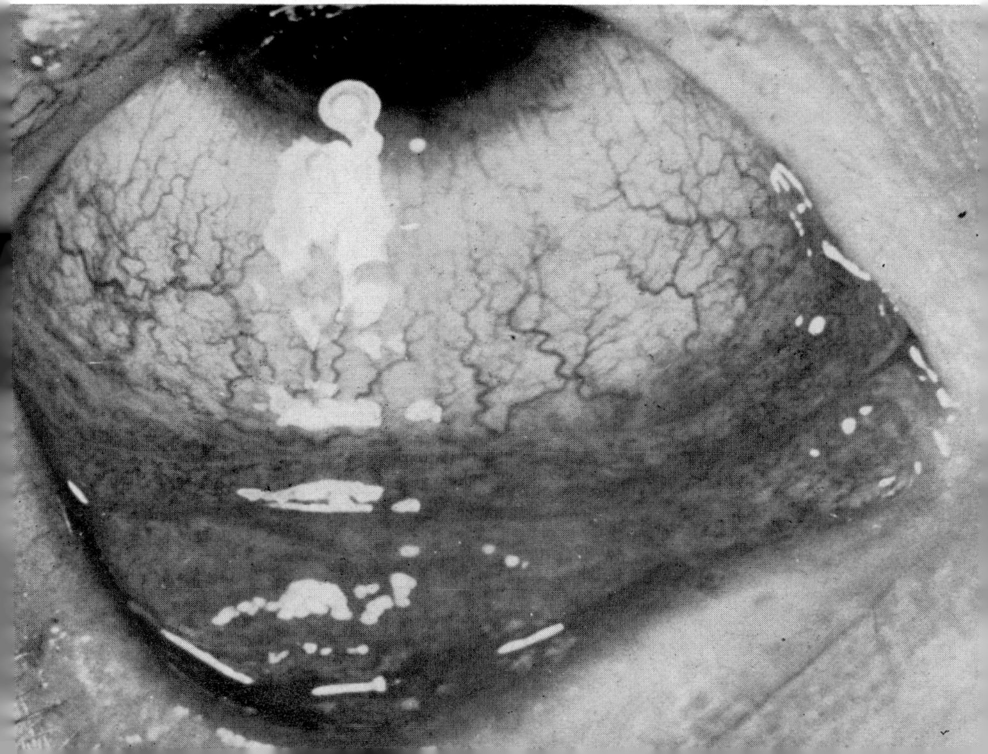

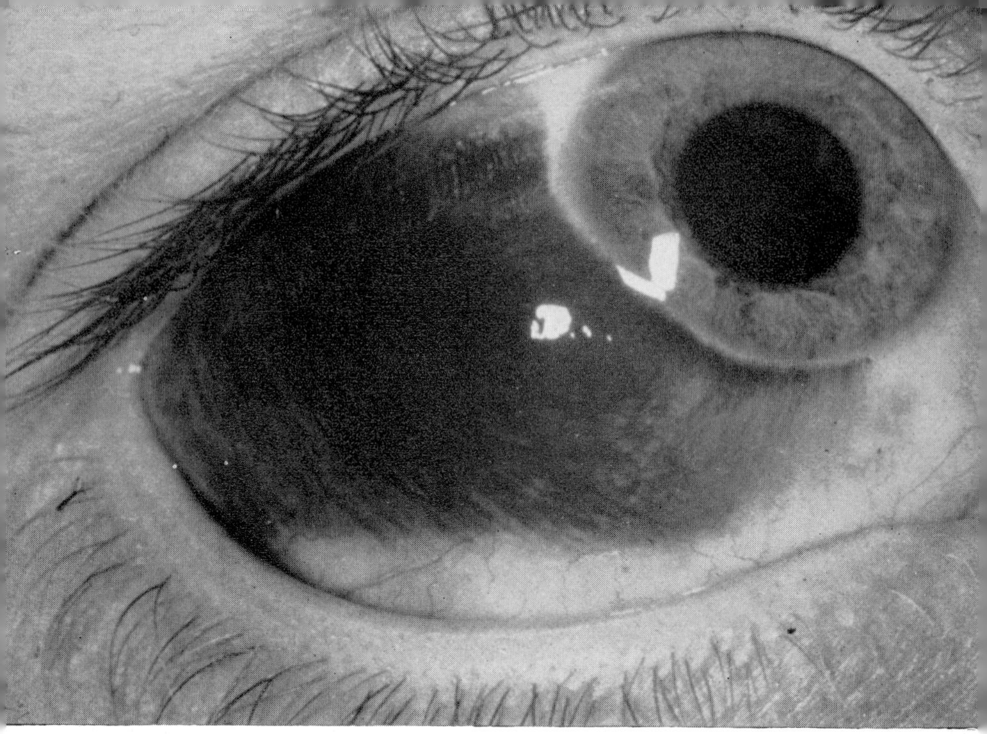

PLATE 3 Subconjunctival haemorrhage

PLATE 4 Anterior uveitis with posterior synechiae at 2 o'clock

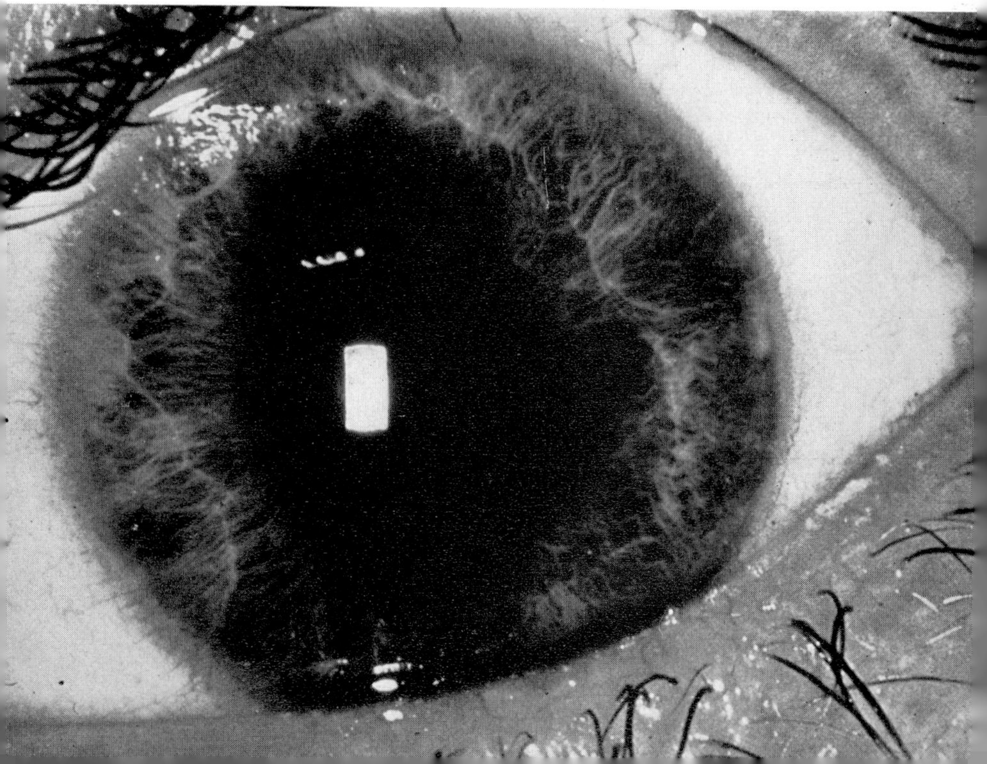

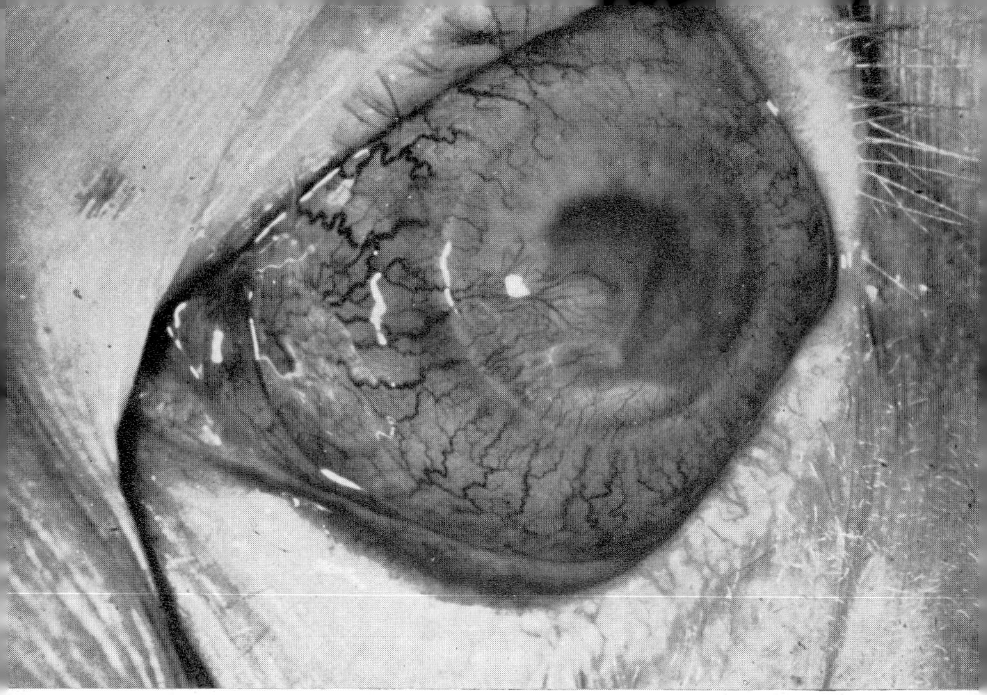

PLATE 5 Hypopyon ulcer with ciliary injection

PLATE 6 Fundus showing haemorrhages and exudates

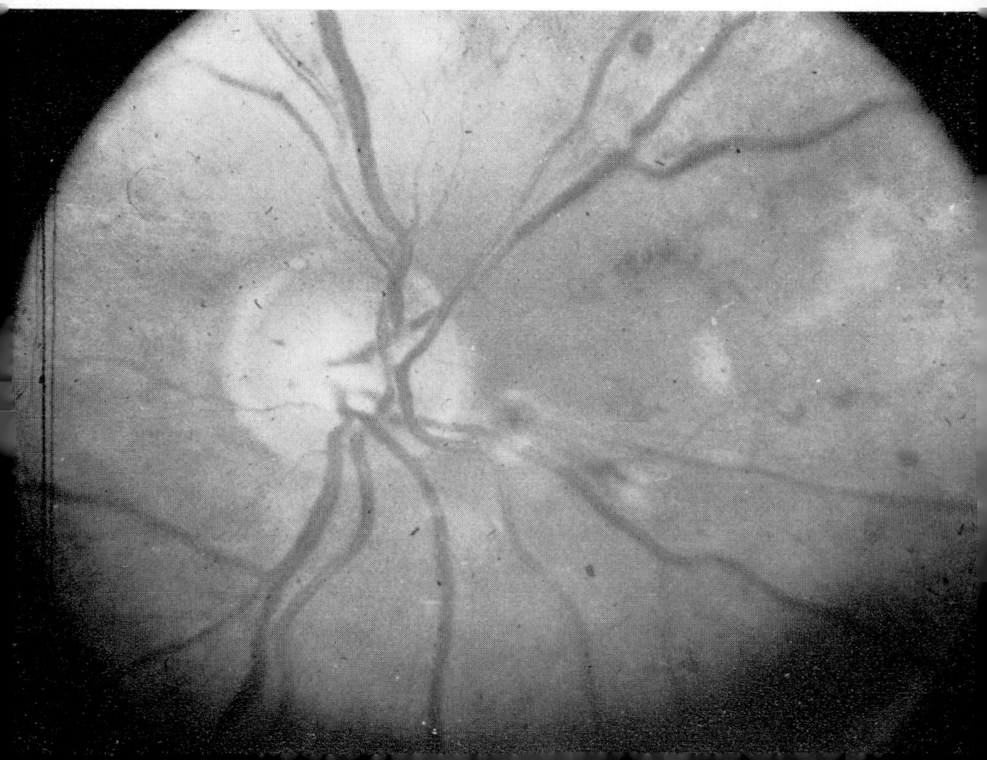

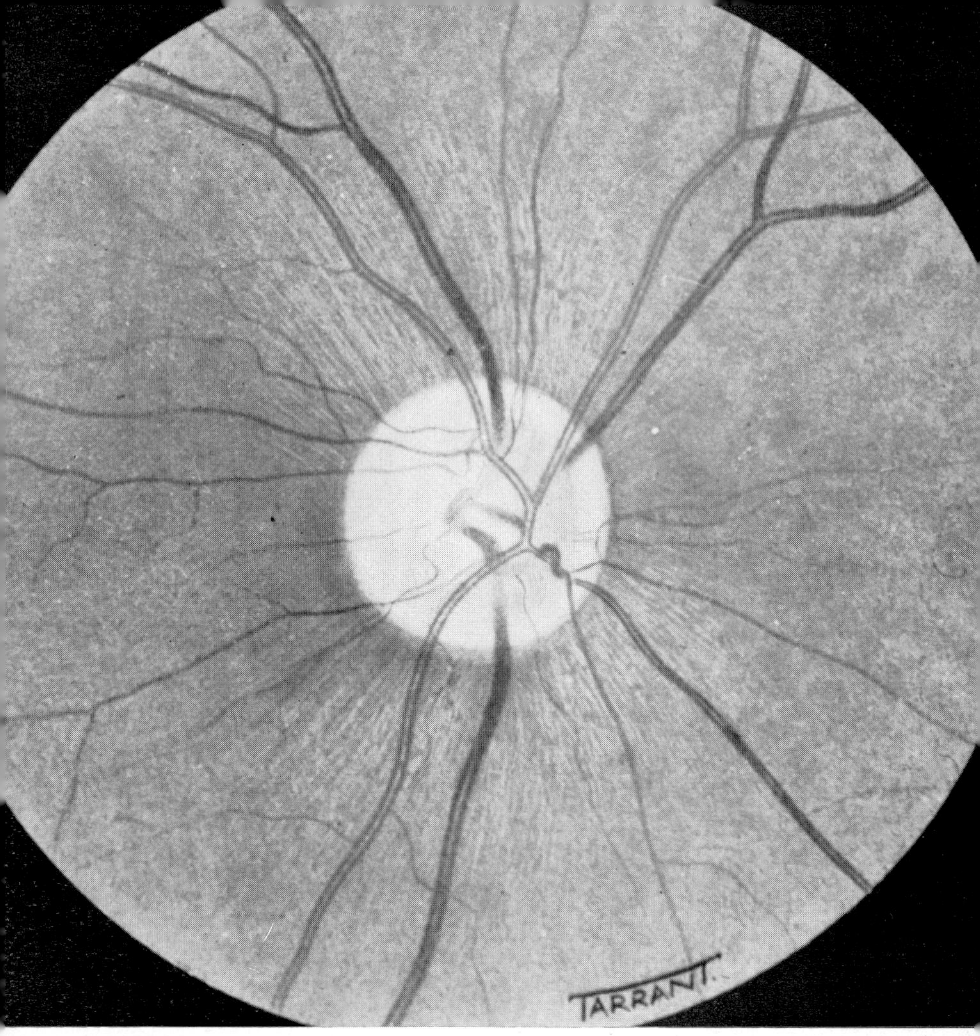

PLATE 7 Normal fundus showing optic papilla and retinal vessels

Neurofibromatosis

This tumour may present in the choroid as part of the manifestations of more widespread neurofibromatosis (von Recklinghausen's disease).

Benign Melanoma

This tumour appears as a slate-grey mass situated deep to the retina. Its size tends to remain static and does not give any deterioration of vision. After middle age a malignant change may occur with the onset of serous detachment of the retina.

Malignant

Malignant Melanoma

This tumour may occur anywhere in the uvea to which it is initially confined but from which it may invade adjacent tissues or even spread outside the eyeball.

Microscopically, the tumour consists of round or spindle cells with a variable admixture of melanin and reticulin which are infiltrated by thin-walled blood spaces.

The initial stages may be asymptomatic unless it involves the macular area when visual disturbances appear.

Malignant melanomata of the iris present as a mass which gradually increases in size and gives distortion of the pupil. The tumour which is usually pigmented may give rise to blurring of vision which may be because an extravasation of blood occurs from it into the anterior chamber or because of secondary glaucoma.

Melanomata of the choroid present a dark coloration with a raised mass over which the retina is elevated or stretched. Fluid from the tumour area tends to gravitate towards the dependent lower fundus where a remote retinal separation appears. Haemorrhages and pigment upset may be visible on the surface of the tumour. Transillumination reveals a shadow corresponding to the melanoma. Extraocular spread may be direct via the scleral channels or haematogenous along the blood spaces—metastasis typically being to the liver. Occasionally a secondary glaucoma results.

TREATMENT

Enucleation of the eyeball containing the malignant melanoma would seem to be the treatment of choice. But, when there is spread into the orbit, exenteration may be preferable. It is important, however, to remember that enucleation does not necessarily increase the expectancy of life because metastasis may occur at any time beforehand. Radioactive cobalt (Co-60) attached to the sclera overlying the neoplasm may give good results as, indeed, does excision of the more accessible ones (e.g. partial choroidectomy or iridocyclectomy).

Metastatic Tumours

Metastatic spread to the uvea of carcinomata of the breast, lung, prostate and stomach occurs. These intraocular deposits are usually in the posterior choroid. By the time secondaries are observed in the eye, metastasis is also present elsewhere thus making enucleation usually unjustifiable.

7 *DISEASES OF THE LENS*

ANATOMY

The lens develops from ectodermal cells which thicken and separate from the adjacent cells to come between the margins of the secondary optic vesicle.

The healthy adult lens is transparent and biconvex while the anterior surface is less convex than the posterior. It is held in position between the iris and vitreous by the suspensory ligament which not only gains attachment to the equator of the lens but also to its anterior and posterior surfaces.

The lens capsule is the homogeneous outer covering of the lens. The epithelium extends over the anterior part of the lens but towards the equator of the lens the epithelial cells become transformed into lens fibres. These form the bulk of the lens and some of the fibres gain attachment to homogeneous 'lines' known as lens sutures. The older fibres are situated towards the centre of the lens called the nucleus while the younger fibres are peripheral—in the cortex. The lens is avascular and derives its nourishment from the aqueous bathing it.

CONGENITAL ABNORMALITIES

Lenticonus

This is the name given to an excessive bowing of the anterior or posterior poles of the lens. Irregular refraction and high myopia are common.

Coloboma

A localised notching of the lens usually situated in its lower part is known as a coloboma. Lenticular opacities are also frequently coincidental.

Ectopia Lentis

Maldevelopment of some fibres of the suspensory ligament may result in displacement of the lens. The lens is then more spherical and therefore more myopic. This condition, usually bilateral, is rare and the lens may not support the iris thus making the iris tremulous (iridodonesis).

Ectopia lentis may occur as an isolated entity but sometimes in addition to arachnodactyly, kyphosis, necrosis of the wall of the aorta and infantilism, the syndrome being called Marfan's syndrome.

In some cases, it is possible to fit spectacles which improve vision but with others it may be necessary to extract the lens.

CATARACT

Cataract is the term used for opacification of the lens. Focal illumination shows up the white opacities which may be situated in different parts of the lens but, on ophthalmoscopy, they appear as dark opacities. As opacification progresses, the lens becomes less transparent and the red reflex from the fundus decreases. Eventually, the whole lens is opaque and easily seen on illuminating the pupillary area.

Cataract may be conveniently described in the following groups.

1 Congenital Cataract

This is the term reserved for opacification of the lens present at birth, and described according to the part of the lens affected.

(a) *Anterior polar cataract*

This small white opacity of the lens is situated at its anterior pole and may sometimes assume a pyramidal shape although it is more commonly round. Sometimes, the cataract arises from maldevelopment of the anterior segment. Like many developmental or congenital cataracts, it is frequently bilateral. When this cataract appears after birth, it originates from perforation of the cornea, either ulceration or injury, thus allowing the cornea and lens to come into contact. The circumscribed lens opacity does not usually reduce vision.

(b) *Posterior polar cataract*

This opacity arises as a result of maldevelopment due to persistence of the primitive nourishing (hyaloid) artery.

(c) *Lamellar or Zonular Cataract*

This is probably the most common congenital cataract in which the fine opacities are restricted to a narrow zone around the nucleus. This cataract is often bilateral. The dust-like opacification may be more dense at its periphery from which white linear opacities project into the transparent surrounding cortex. The visual upset depends on the density of the cataract.

(d) *Coronary cataract* is characterised by the presence of pear-shaped or club-like opacities in the cortex of the lens. Sometimes the opacities are dust-like, have a bluish colour and rarely reduce vision.

Rubella Cataract

Rubella or German Measles during the second and third months of pregnancy is particularly liable to cause cataract in the foetus. The cataract tends to be not only bilateral but also extensive. At the same time, rubella may attack the retina giving a pigmentary degeneration referred to as rubella retinopathy.

2 Senile Cataract

This is the commonest form of cataract, rarely seen before the age of forty but which is more frequent in succeeding decades. In some pedigrees, cataract seems to occur in succeeding generations whereas in others it is sporadic.

Two main forms of senile cataract predominate: one with opacities principally situated in the nucleus (nuclear) and the other in the cortex. In nuclear sclerosis there is a gradual hardening of the lens nucleus which increases myopia. This sclerosis progresses incipiently into a frank opacification in the central part of the lens. Despite the nuclear changes, the surrounding cortex is very often clear.

Where the cortex becomes opacified (cortical cataract), the nucleus is clear at least in the early stages. As the cataract spreads throughout the cortex vision becomes more and more impaired. Dilatation of the pupil reveals the greyish opacities to be radially arranged and cuneiform in shape (wedge-shaped), the wider end is peripheral (see Fig. 14). More rarely, the opacities are grouped in the posterior

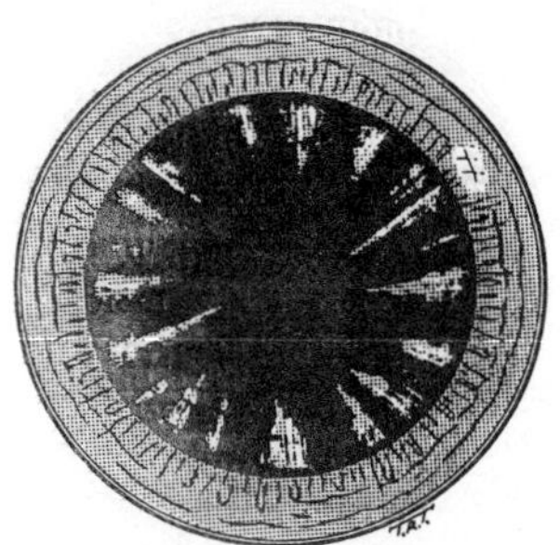

FIG 14 Cuneiform cataract

cortex (cupuliform cataract). The lens normally increases in size because of fluid absorption, but as the cataract matures much of the fluid is lost as the lens then becomes more opaque. The eye, however, retains at least perception of light provided no other pathology is present. Occasionally, the lens assumes a dark brown colour as it shrinks. Sometimes the cortex liquefies and the solid nucleus sinks down towards the capsule (Morgagnian cataract); such a cataract is hypermature.

Hypermaturity should be avoided by extracting the lens because it may (a) become dislocated into the vitreous, (b) release lens substance through a capsular deficiency and give rise to secondary glaucoma (phacolytic), (c) irritate the uvea—lens induced uveitis. While the lens matures, fluid absorption may be so great that the increased size of the lens pushes the iris forwards against the filtration spaces so precipitating glaucoma.

3 Traumatic Cataract

This type of cataract follows direct injury to the lens capsule e.g. penetrating injury. Sometimes a blunt injury to the eye may rupture the lens capsule and produce a concussion cataract. Aqueous quickly permeates through the breach in the capsule and the lens not only becomes opaque but swells, while some of the swollen lens contents protrude from the capsular tear.

In some the lens substance absorbs and leaves only capsular remnants in the pupillary area but in others the lens protein excites a uveitis.

4 Complicated Cataract

This is subsequent to other disease in the eye e.g. uveitis, glaucoma, retinal detachment. The cataract has a characteristic polychromatic lustre as it extends in the posterior cortex.

5 Irradiation Cataract

This follows exposure to radium or X-rays, and slowly spreads from the posterior cortex where it originates. Extraction may be required after a few years when the entire lens is opaque.

6 Diabetic Cataract

Pure diabetic cataract is seen in the young. When diabetes mellitus occurs in the aged, the lens changes tend to be senile in nature without the distinguishing features of a diabetic cataract. The incidence and progress of lens changes in the elderly appear to be greater when diabetes is also present.

Fine white dust-like subcapsular opacities (rather like a snow-storm) in both eyes characterise diabetic cataracts in the young. Sometimes they have a polychromatic lustre. If the diabetes is quickly controlled the opacities may remain static and not appreciably impair vision, but ill-regulated diabetes promotes increasing opacification.

A hyperglycaemia causes a swing of the refraction towards increasing myopia while hypoglycaemia makes the eye more hypermetropic.

Cataract may accompany other endocrine upsets e.g. hypoparathyroidism and hypothyroidism. Cataract may arise with various skin disorders, toxins, mongolism, myotonic dystrophy and retinitis pigmentosa.

TREATMENT OF CATARACT

It is important to examine both eyes thoroughly before deciding whether or not to operate for cataract. The indications for surgery are outside the scope of this book, but the aim of surgery should be to improve the visual acuity.

In some cases of nuclear cataract, it may be possible to improve vision to tolerable levels by changing the spectacle correction. This, however, is usually only a temporary measure. In nuclear cataract, dilatation of the pupil may allow improvement of vision.

It may be necessary to treat any existing disease e.g. diabetes, uveitis or glaucoma before embarking on surgery.

Discission

In children a discission may often be the operation of choice. The anterior lens capsule is opened with a discission needle, thus permitting aqueous to enter the lens. The lens matter then swells up and eventually absorbs satisfactorily in many cases. In others the lens matter gathers in the filtration spaces and causes raised intraocular tension. This tension may be controlled by oral acetazolamide while the lens particles spontaneously absorb or be relieved by irrigation of the anterior chamber thus washing out the lens matter.

This operation leaves the posterior lens capsule within the pupil and it is often sufficiently transparent to permit good vision. If the capsular remnants are too dense they can be needled so that a gap is left through which clear vision is possible.

Extracapsular Extraction

In this operation the eye is opened at or near the limbus above, and the anterior lens capsule incised or even largely removed to allow expression of most of the lens fibres. Much of any remaining lens matter may be removed by irrigation. An iridectomy, either peripheral or broad, is desirable to permit the flow of aqueous from posterior to anterior chambers (this is because posterior synechiae between the iris and capsular remnants may obstruct the normal flow of aqueous through the pupil). Subsequent needling of the capsular membrane some weeks or months later may be needed to provide good vision.

Intracapsular Extraction

A limbal incision is made above (rarely below) and an iridectomy or iridotomy fashioned. The lens is then extracted within its capsule either by simple expression, by capsule forceps, by erisophake suction or by cryoextraction. Alphachymotrypsin solution instilled behind the iris permits digestion of zonular fibres thus facilitating their early rupture and the removal of the entire lens.

At the time of the operation, severe haemorrhage may occur from the choroid (expulsive haemorrhage) and lead to extrusion of much of the contents of the eyeball. Such an eye is in most cases visually useless but occasionally useful vision may still remain after the blood is absorbed. Blood may gather in the anterior chamber at or after operation. In the majority of cases, this hyphema absorbs without complication.

Prolapse of the iris through the section may follow operation. This requires surgical correction.

Occasionally, vitreous loss occurs during operation. In most cases this is not serious, but sometimes it is followed by changes directly attributable to this vitreous loss e.g. corneal dystrophy, retinal detachment or glaucoma.

Pathogenic organisms may enter the eye at the time of operation and if this endophthalmitis is even suspected, urgent treatment with antibiotics must be immediately instituted.

DISLOCATION OF THE LENS

This arises as a developmental anomaly or following trauma. Dislocation is rarely seen in other conditions e.g. congenital glaucoma. The dislocation may be partial (subluxation) or complete, and displacement is either anterior or posterior.

Anterior dislocation usually tends to cause visual blurring because of the lens displacement and because of the tilting of the lens. An anteriorly displaced lens is more easily removed because of its accessibility. It is therefore desirable to obtain pupillary miosis if the lens is anterior to the pupil so that the lens does not readily fall posteriorly.

Posterior dislocation may give little visual upset if the lens does not lie in the visual axis. If the lens is outside this axis, an aphakic spectacle correction may well give good vision. In other patients, however, the lens lies in the vitreous, or on the retina or ciliary body. Positioning on the latter sites may result in retinal detachment or glaucoma.

The treatment of dislocation of the lens in most cases is removal of the lens, but the results are sometimes disappointing.

8 *DISORDERS OF THE VITREOUS*

ANATOMY

The vitreous is a transparent, colourless gel which occupies much of the posterior part of the eye behind the lens. The periphery of the vitreous is condensed to form an equally transparent hyaloid membrane. The protein of the vitreous attracts water and becomes arranged in sheaths. Apart from residual protein a polysaccharide called hyaluronic acid is present in the vitreous where this acid plays a fundamental part in the maintenance of its transparency. Normal vitreous is devoid of blood vessels and is nourished from the surrounding structures by permeation.

CONGENITAL ABNORMALITIES

Persistent Hyaloid Artery

The foetal lens is nourished in part by an artery which passes from the optic disc through the vitreous to the lens. This artery, which normally disappears as pregnancy approaches full-time, may persist in post-natal life when a lens opacity is often present nasal to the posterior pole of the lens. In others persistence of the foetal artery is more marked and appears as a fibro-vascular cord in the vitreous.

Persistent Hyperplastic Vitreous

A mass of vascularised tissue is present in the anterior vitreous after birth. The ciliary processes become atrophic and elongated while the anterior chamber is shallow and the retina becomes detached. Uveitis and glaucoma (secondary) are likely sequelae.

DISEASES OF THE VITREOUS

Muscae Volitantes

This is the term used when fine opacities appear in the vitreous and result from congenital abnormalities or changes in the protein of the vitreous. They cause the patient to see greyish or dark spots in front of the affected eye or eyes, particularly when the illumination is good or on looking at a bright background. The spots move with changes in the position of the eyes but do not affect vision. No treatment is known to influence the absorption of muscae volitantes.

Synchisis Scintillans

This usually unilateral degeneration of the vitreous often follows haemorrhage into the vitreous or uveitis. There are numerous fine cholesterol crystals in the fluid vitreous which move with ocular movements but which rarely cause visual symptoms. These crystals persist in great numbers but do not require treatment.

Asteroid Hyalitis

This degeneration of the vitreous appears in the elderly, seldom causes visual upset and does not require treatment. The white opacities consist of calcium soaps.

Vitreous opacities may also arise in conjunction with uveitis, from retinal haemorrhage with leakage of blood cells into the vitreous, and in detachment of the retina.

Vitreous Detachment

In old age the vitreous may shrink and become separated from the retina posteriorly. Patients with this vitreous detachment observe spots in front of the affected eye. Vision is generally good.

Vitreous Haemorrhage

Haemorrhage into the vitreous may occur from vessels in the retina, uvea or even from abnormal vessels in the vitreous itself.

Occasionally, bleeding from the retina may not break into the vitreous but be contained between the internal limiting layer of the retina and the hyaloid membrane. Such a haemorrhage is known as preretinal and has a curved outline with a linear horizontal upper edge.

When bleeding is more extensive, the blood cells pass into the vitreous which then becomes tinted red. Vision is often reduced.

Smaller vitreous haemorrhages absorb satisfactorily but in larger ones with much tissue tearing there is an attempt to organise the haemorrhage. This results in a fibrovascular proliferation into the vitreous from the torn retina (retinitis proliferans) in an attempt to organise the blood.The strands of fibrous tissue contract and may pull sufficiently on the retina to detach it (traction retinal detachment).

Vitreous haemorrhage occurs in a wide variety of conditions e.g. following trauma, myopia, hypertension, diabetes, blood dyscrasias, retinal vasculitis and neoplasms.

9 *DISEASES OF THE RETINA*

ANATOMY

The retina is a fine membrane forming the innermost of the three coats of the eyeball and has an important role in visual perception. The retina extends from its anterior extremity, the ora serrata, to the optic disc or papilla, into which the retinal nerve fibrils pass. Healthy retina is transparent but it may become opacified in disease or death. The posterior retina presents a 1–2 mm depression called the macula lutea which has a central area, the fovea centralis. This part of the retina is concerned with maximal visual discrimination and helps one to appreciate detail.

The optic disc or papilla, is about 3 mm nasal to the posterior pole. The central retinal artery and vein enter and leave the eye at the optic disc while the nerve fibrils converge from the retina onto the papilla (optic disc) before making their exit from the eye.

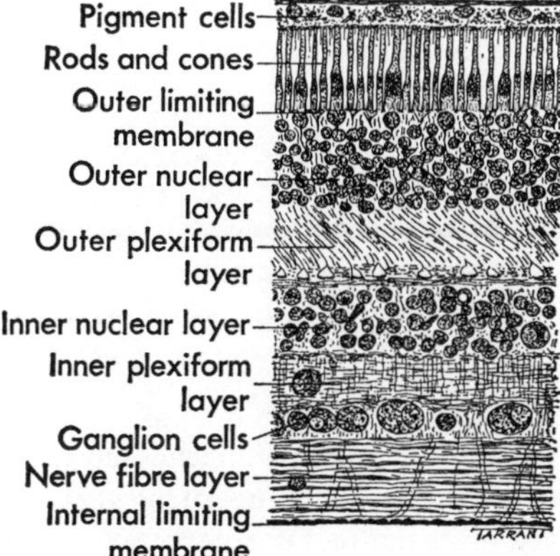

FIG 15 Diagrammatic representation of the structure of the retina

The structure of the retina is graphically shown in Fig. 15 and consists from without inwards of:

(1) Pigment cells (hexagonal epithelium)
(2) Layer of rods and cones (rhodopsin, the visual purple is within the rods)
(3) Outer limiting membrane
(4) Outer nuclear layer (which is made up of the rod and cone nuclei)
(5) Outer plexiform layer (an arborisation of fibres from the nuclear layers)
(6) Inner nuclear layer (bipolar cells which are connecting cells between the rods and cones and the ganglion cells)
(7) Inner plexiform layer (an arborisation of fibres from the bipolar and the ganglion cells)
(8) Ganglion cell layer

(9) Nerve fibre layer which consists of the axons of the ganglion cells; the axonal fibres converge on the optic papilla to pass further along the optic nerve to the brain

(10) The internal limiting membrane

The outer layers are nourished by diffusion from the choroid but the inner layers of the retina are supplied by the retinal artery which itself is an end artery and does not anastomose with the ciliary vessels.

CONGENITAL ABNORMALITIES

Opaque Nerve Fibres

Medullation of the optic nerve is normally present as far as the lamina cribrosa. Sometimes medullation extends further along the nerve into the retina when these medullated fibres (opaque nerve fibres) present a white fluffy patch near the optic disc. Apart from a scotoma (visual field defect) corresponding with the area of opaque nerve fibres no visual upset is experienced.

Coloboma

This congenital malformation is usually situated inferonasally where the choroid and retina have failed to develop. Vision in the affected area is usually also defective. The defect is due to incomplete fusion of the edges of the optic vesicle during foetal life.

Albinism

In this condition there is defective development of pigment throughout the body. The iris of the eye is blue while the blood vessels of the eye impart a red or pink colour. There is also photophobia, nystagmus and defective vision.

Retrolental Fibroplasia

This is found almost exclusively in premature children who have been exposed to excessive oxygen (more than 30%) immediately after birth. The condition is bilateral and the oxygen gives rise to vasoconstriction during oxygen administration, but vessel proliferation appears on withdrawal of oxygen. After an initial greyish coloration of the peripheral retina, vascularised tissue with haemorrhages is visible behind the lens. Contracture of this tissue may give rise to retinal detachment and poor vision. Neovascularisation may appear on the iris and even secondary glaucoma can supervene. Treatment is essentially prophylactic, namely, the avoidance of excessive oxygen.

Pigmentary Retinopathy

This usually follows maternal infections such as syphilis and rubella during the first three months of pregnancy. The condition is bilateral and characterised by a pigmentary mottling in the fundi. If the macula is involved there is a diminution of vision.

Retinal Dysplasia

In this bilateral condition there is maldevelopment of the retina which has a greyish colour. The retina becomes detached and may adhere to the posterior surface of the lens. Microphthalmos is usually present and the anterior chambers are shallow. Treatment is of no avail.

INJURIES

Commotio Retinae

Oedema of the retina characterises this condition which follows a blow to the eye. The affected area of the retina is pale and swelling of the odematous retina is evident, while occasional haemorrhages may also be visible in this traumatised retina. The commotio retinae may be at the site of the injury or a contrecoup oedema may present at the macula. The commotio generally resolves without apparent defect, but pigmentary upset may be visible in the retina on absorption of the oedema while in others cystic change may supervene. Vision is usually good unless there is a marked disturbance of macular function. Rest is the most satisfactory therapy.

Retinal Haemorrhage

Haemorrhage may follow either blunt or penetrating injury to the eye and the size of the haemorrhage varies greatly. A marked effusion of blood may break from the retina into the vitreous.

Detachment of the Retina

This may follow trauma to the retina, particularly where there is a breach of retinal tissue as in perforating injuries.

Solar Retinopathy

Direct gazing at the sun or an eclipse of the sun with the unprotected eye may produce a burn of the retina. There is initial retinal oedema at the macular area but this oedema absorbs and is replaced by pigmentary disturbance. Vision is impaired and there is a central scotoma.

INFLAMMATION OF THE RETINA

Inflammation of the retina (retinitis) is seldom restricted to the retina itself but often also involves the choroid (choroidoretinitis).

Metastatic Retinitis

An infected embolus may be transported along the central retinal artery and become impacted in the retinal arteriole where a localised inflammatory reaction starts. There is a circumscribed haziness in the retina with one or two small haemorrhages. The inflammation destroys the neural elements and this may give a localised scotoma or, if the nerve fibres are also involved, a sectorial defect arises. Virulent organisms will produce sepsis which spreads and gives rise to panophthalmitis. In milder infections some inflammatory cells from the retina pass into the vitreous and make it cloudy. Treatment is adequate systemic antibiotic therapy.

Exudative Retinitis (Coat's Disease)

This condition usually occurs in male children between five and twenty years of age. It is typically unilateral. The lesion is situated in the region of the posterior pole where there are intraretinal haemorrhage and exudation. Pathologically, there is a retinal telangiectasia and some extravasation which produces retinal detachment. Because of its chronicity, there are cholesterol crystals in the extravasion. The visual acuity is grossly impaired and treatment is of no avail because of its inefficacy.

Retinal Vasculitis

This is the name given to inflammation of the retinal veins and arteries. Histologically, there is a perivascular infiltration by white cells from the bloodstream. It occurs in young adults, particularly males, who are often otherwise apparently healthy. Vision tends to be good to begin with because the major lesions are in the peripheral retina where calibre variations, haemorrhage and vascular occlusions are found. The retinal haemorrhage may be large and extend into the vitreous. Although remissions are the rule, relapses also occur and sometimes massive vitreous haemorrhage leaves marked visual impairment. Organising fibrovascular bands grow from the diseased retina into the vitreous in an endeavour to organise the haemorrhage—retinitis proliferans.

Rarely, the vasculitis involves the retinal vessels at the optic disc. Here, there is marked engorgement of the retinal veins throughout their distribution. Oedema is present at the optic disc and at the macula.

Systemic steroids often give a marked improvement in the condition but sometimes light coagulation is applied to the diseased vessels.

Central Serous Retinopathy

Macular oedema and maintenance of adequate vision are present in this condition usually found in young adults. The visual acuity is only slightly reduced and there is some distortion of images in addition to altered colour appreciation. Fluorescein photography may reveal a leakage from one of the retinal arterioles. Sealing of this breach in the arterioles is followed by absorption of the macular oedema. Spontaneous resolution is usual in a few weeks but pigmentary mottling in the macular area may be permanent.

Light coagulation applied to the area of the vascular leak may seal the breach but systemic steroids may aid spontaneous resolution.

VASCULAR DISORDERS

Hyperaemia may involve the arteries and/or veins which become engorged and tortuous.

Severe anaemia, on the other hand, frequently results in pallor of the fundus and attenuated retinal arterioles.

In the blood dyscrasias, the retinal veins are dilated and retinal haemorrhages are of varying number.

RETINOPATHY

Atheroma

This lipoid degeneration of the intima (or innermost coat) of an artery may, in the case of the retinal artery, lead to partial or total occlusion of the vessel lumen. The affected vessel assumes a white coloration.

Arteriolar Sclerosis

In essential hypertension there is a thickening of the intima which later involves the entire vessel wall which appears narrowed and conveys a decreased volume of blood.

Hypertensive Retinopathy

In the early stages the retinal arteries are narrowed, pale and straight while the veins are engorged distal to the arteriovenous crossings. Later the thickened arterial walls are less translucent and the retinal veins become concealed at the arteriovenous junctions. The circulating blood columns in the diseased arterioles are irregular. As the hypertension continues, a replacement fibrosis appears in the arterial wall and the vessel is irregularly irregular besides assuming a copper wire coloration. In severe hypertension these changes are more marked and the circulating blood is reduced because of increasing degeneration of the vessel wall. Small haemorrhages appear in the posterior retina and they often have a striate appearance because of their presence between the nerve fibrils. Haemorrhages may sometimes be large and hard white exudates occur in the posterior fundus (Plate 6). In addition, cotton wool exudates (soft and white) appear in the superficial retinal areas affected by arteriolar occlusion. Oedema of the optic disc and perimacular area may also occur.

Toxaemic Retinopathy

In pre-eclampsia of pregnancy hypertension is also manifest. The retinal arterioles become narrowed and constricted while retinal and papillary oedema may be found in addition to cotton-wool exudates and haemorrhages. Occasionally the features of malignant hypertension appear, and there may even be an exudative detachment of the inferior retina. As the toxaemia of pregnancy subsides, the detachment resolves. The retinal arterioles, on the other hand, exhibit some sclerosis and pigmentary upset of the retina persists if the hypertension continues.

Diabetic Retinopathy

Diabetic retinopathy occurs more commonly in elderly patients who have suffered from diabetes mellitus for many years. The retinopathy may be present even when the diabetes mellitus is well controlled. It is almost always bilateral.

The earliest ophthalmoscopic appearance is engorgement of the retinal veins and capillary hyperaemia. Small saccular dilatations or microaneurysms then appear at the venous ends of the retinal capillaries and are recognisable as small red dots in the retina. They may be confused in appearance with small retinal haemorrhages but microaneurysms persist in contrast to haemorrhages of similar size which tend to absorb. Later, blot haemorrhages are evident in the deeper layers of the retina as a result of the diapedesis from the degenerate retinal vessels. White exudates are then visible in the retina and as they become more numerous they tend to agglomerate.

Haemorrhage may be more extensive and break from the retina into the vitreous. Attempts to organise this haemorrhage may result in retinitis proliferans, a fibrovascular proliferation from the retina into the vitreous. In others a delicate network of fine new vessels may form in the vitreous-rete mirabile. Unfortunately the fibrovascular tissue contracts and may cause detachment of the retina.

Arteriosclerosis is often present with diabetic retinopathy in the elderly, and impaired blood supply may give rise to optic atrophy. In the young diabetic, retinal lipaemia may be seen and the excessive circulating fat in the blood gives a yellowish pallor to the retinal vessels.

Because of the tendency for the retinopathy to involve the macular area at an early stage, visual deterioration may well be an early feature.

Treatment

It is desirable to assiduously control the diabetes mellitus in the hope of alleviating the deterioration. It has been suggested that oral Atromid delays the progress of the fundus changes but this is not yet widely accepted. On the other hand, beneficial results have followed ablation of the pituitary or its destruction by Yttrium implants (a radioactive implant).

Obstruction of the Central Retinal Artery

Obstruction of the central retinal artery may arise as a result of (1) Embolism (from the impaction in the artery of a fragment of an intracardiac vegetation); (2) Thrombosis (e.g. due to changes in the vessel wall); (3) Spasm (hypertonus of the arterial wall). Vision may be lost entirely, suddenly and permanently (amaurosis) but sometimes forewarning may be in the nature of transient attacks of blurred vision. A small fragment of vision may be retained when some blood is passed to the retina via the collateral circulation of the cilioretinal artery.

Soon after occlusion of the central retinal artery, the retina becomes whitish due to the coagulative necrosis of the ischaemic inner layers of the retina. The fovea, in contrast, maintains a bright red colour. The retinal arterioles are extremely attenuated or obliterated while the direct pupillary response to light is very sluggish or absent. The obliterated retinal arteries stand out prominently as white chords but if some blood passes along them they may regain a red tint. Pigmentary mottling appears at the macula while some weeks after the onset of the occlusion, atrophy of the optic disc is evident.

If only one of the branches of the retinal artery is occluded, the ischaemic degeneration is limited to the area of retina supplied by the vessels and the sector of defective vision corresponds to that same part of the retina.

TREATMENT

Only occasionally is treatment successful, but early administration of retrobulbar tolazoline or acetylcholine may help together with paracentesis.

Giant-cell Arteritis

Giant-cell arteritis is a condition in which there are widespread inflammatory foci in the vessel wall which gives rise to localised encroachment of the lumen. This may be so marked that there is occlusion of the central retinal artery. The condition is more common over the age of 60 years, when sudden loss of vision and headache are striking features. The erythrocyte sedimentation rate is raised. If systemic steroids are administered at an early stage, improvement in vision sometimes occurs but these steroids will be of value in minimising a possible occlusion of the fellow artery.

Post-haemorrhagic Amaurosis

Post-haemorrhagic amaurosis may sometimes follow marked and recurrent bleeding from the gastrointestinal tract. The fundus in these cases is pale due to the ischaemia, while retinal haemorrhages and exudates may appear in addition to oedema of the optic disc. Immediate transfusion of blood may lessen the residual visual defect by restoring normal circulating blood.

Thrombosis of the Central Retinal Vein

This may arise in the vein at the lamina cribrosa, or in one of the tributaries of the central retinal vein (i.e. a partial occlusion).

Thrombosis of the vein may occur in glaucoma, also when a sclerosed artery unduly compresses the vein, in the presence of retinal vasculitis and occasionally in blood dyscrasias.

The affected veins are grossly engorged and numerous haemorrhages are present along the course of the affected vessel. New vessels form in the area affected by the thrombosis and serve as a delicate anastomosing network which serves to partially restore the circulation.

During the succeeding months, the retinal haemorrhages absorb, but new vessels grow on the iris (about three months after the thrombosis) and course into the spaces of the filtration angle thereby blocking them and causing thrombotic glaucoma.

Treatment is often disappointing but should be directed towards the underlying cause. Anticoagulants are sometimes used.

PRIMARY RETINAL DEGENERATIONS

Heredomacular Degeneration

The onset may vary with regard to age, hence the tendency to refer to it as congenital, infantile, juvenile, adolescent, adult and senile forms. The initial features are pigmentary mottling at the maculae accompanied by a diminution of central vision. The vision may be satisfactory for some years but eventually it steadily decreases. The visual defect is only for central vision involving the macula, thus the patient retains peripheral vision and should never become blind. Telescopic spectacles or a magnifying glass are the only known means of improving vision in some.

Retinitis Pigmentosa

This is a primary retinal degeneration initially involving the pigment epithelium and the rods and cones. The bilateral degeneration is inevitably progressive as it runs a chronic course. It is an inherited disease occurring more frequently in males.

The earliest manifestations of the disease occur in adolescence with the onset of night blindness. There is a degeneration of the equatorial part of the retina which produces an annular scotoma. Unfortunately this scotoma gradually enlarges to leave only a small central island of vision (corresponding to the macular area). The retention of this is compatible with good central vision without a peripheral field of vision. In mid-life even this may be eroded and then vision markedly falls.

Ophthalmoscopically, the degenerate pigment of the retina is aggregated into somewhat stellate-like lumps resembling bone corpuscles while the pigment may sheath the retinal vessels. The retinal arterioles are markedly attenuated and thus not so readily visible in the fundus which also has an atrophic optic disc of waxy yellow colour. Occasionally, a pigment upset is not a prominent feature of the degeneration—*degeneratio sine pigmento*. An additional impediment to vision is the late onset of a genetically linked posterior polar cataract. The cataractous lens may be extracted without undue difficulty but other treatment is of no avail.

Amaurotic Family Idiocy

This progressive degeneration of the ganglion cells not only of the retina but also of the central nervous system is usually confined to the Jewish race. Ophthalmoscopically, the retina appears to have a cherry-red spot at the macula with a large surrounding pale halo, while the optic disc is atrophic and the retinal arterioles are attenuated. Vision is markedly diminished and a fatal termination is usual in two years.

Cerebro-macular Degeneration

This degeneration of the central nervous system and the macular regions of both maculae is familial in origin and commences in the earlier years of life. There is a pigmentary upset at the macula and a progressive visual failure before death.

Detachment of the Retina

In this condition, there is a breach in the retinal tissues whereby fluid accumulates between the layer of rods and cones and the pigment epithelium of the retina.

The causal rupture may take various forms: (1) a tear or hole and (2) a dialysis. The former tend to be peripheral and occur more commonly in myopic eyes or in the presence of peripheral areas of degeneration. The retinal dialysis usually follows previous blunt injury to the eye and rupture of a retinal cyst.

The hole or breach in the retina may be present for a short period before giving rise to retinal separation. Sometimes, the onset of a large tear is heralded by the appearance of a vitreous haemorrhage because the tear has also ruptured the retinal vessels coursing across it. As the retina detaches, it assumes a greyish coloration and the accumulation of subretinal fluid gives the detached retina a wavy appearance with darkened retinal vessels undulating over it (Fig. 16).

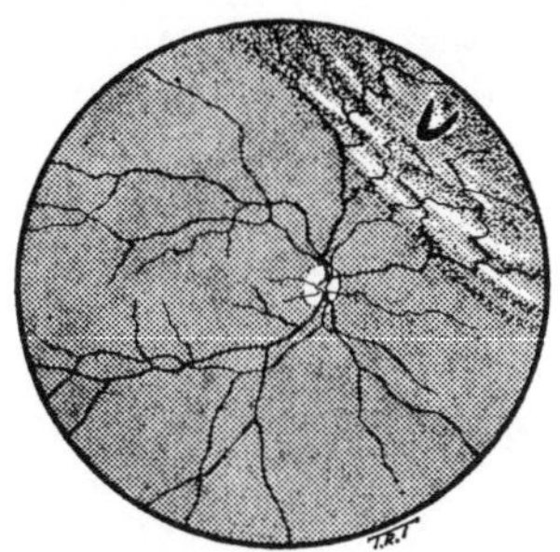

FIG 16 U-shaped tear of the retina

A scotoma corresponding to the detached retina is demonstrable and once the macula becomes detached vision is poor.

TREATMENT

A simple break with little or no subretinal fluid may be sealed by light coagulation or cryosurgery. Extensive accumulations of subretinal fluid require a shortening operation of the eyeball and evacuation of the subretinal fluid. The shortening operation may only be segmental or involve cerclage of the eyeball behind the tear.

In a small number of cases, the injection of donor vitreous into the vitreous of the eye with the retinal detachment may retain the retina in good apposition.

Retinal Cysts

These cysts tend to occur in the peripheral retina and at its posterior pole. They may be small and escape notice but others may slowly enlarge. These cysts do not require treatment unless they rupture or enlarge appreciably.

Secondary Detachment of the Retina

Detachment of the retina may be secondary to other changes e.g. inflammation of the uvea, malignant neoplasm of the choroid, toxaemia of pregnancy, etc. The treatment here is that of the underlying cause.

TOXIC AMBLYOPIA

Some substances are liable to directly poison the ganglion cells of the retina thus producing their malfunction. Other toxic substances may give rise to ischaemic atrophy of the retina because of their constricting action on the retinal vessels (this defective blood supply causes malfunction or death of the affected retinal cells). Degeneration of the retinal ganglion cells causes atrophy of the optic nerve.

(1) *Tobacco Amblyopia*

This usually follows the prolonged smoking or ingestion of pipe tobacco. There is an insidious diminution of vision and a scotoma may be demonstrated between fixation and the blind spot—the so-called centrocaecal scotoma.

Improvement in vision may arise from stopping tobacco and administering Neocytamin.

(2) *Alcohol Amblyopia*

The findings are similar to that of tobacco but methyl alcohol may produce permanent damage to the ganglion cells and even blindness.

(3) *Quinine Amblyopia*

Quinine produces a permanent defect of vision which may even result in blindness. The drug causes intense constriction of the retinal arterioles thus giving retinal ischaemia. The optic disc becomes pale and in less severe cases a scotoma may be demonstrated.

(4) *Chloroquine Amblyopia*

Chloroquine has been widely used as a therapeutic agent but in excessive dosage it produces attenuation of the retinal arterioles and pigmentary degeneration in the macular area. A central scotoma is demonstrable.

Nutritional Amblyopia

Malnutrition over a prolonged period may give rise to amblyopia. The deficiency is mainly of Vitamin B and protein. This amblyopia was particularly common among prisoners of war under the Japanese during the last world war.

Vision is impaired and there may be macular oedema which absorbs to be replaced by some pigmentary mottling. Later the optic disc is atrophic and a small dense central scotoma is characteristic.

NEOPLASMS OF THE RETINA

Retinoblastoma

This primary malignant neoplasm of the retina is of congenital origin and usually presents before the age of five. The neoplasm may be bilateral but, if so, the sizes are usually different in each eye. Many cases are sporadic but an hereditary element is also seen.

Histologically, the tumour consists of small round cells with hyperchromatic nuclei distributed in columnar or rosette fashion with a varying admixture of calcium deposition.

The child's parents usually notice, as a presenting feature, a 'cat's eye reflex' within the pupil and, on examination, the fundus is observed to contain a white mass. The mass enlarges slowly and even fragments with 'seedling deposits'. There is little tendency to haemorrhage but retinal detachment may arise or proliferation occurs into the vitreous. In some cases, tumour cells may pass forwards and be deposited in the anterior chamberas a snowy white 'hypopyon'. In others, seedling deposits appear on the iris.

Spread outside the eye is directly along the optic nerve.

Treatment

When the tumour is large, it is desirable to enucleate the eye and to cut the optic nerve as far posteriorly as possible. This may be followed by irradiation. At the same time, a repeated examination of the fellow eye should be carried out to exclude a similar neoplasm in it.

Smaller retinoblastomata may be successfully treated by radioactive cobalt-60 plaques applied to the sclera overlying the mass.

Secondary malignant neoplasms invade the retina by direct spread from the choroid or optic nerve.

10 *DISEASES OF THE OPTIC NERVE*

ANATOMY

The nerve fibres of the optic nerve are medullated and enclosed by a forward prolongation of the meninges (dura mater, arachnoid, and pia) together with circulating cerebrospinal fluid.

Anatomically, the nerve is divided into four portions:

(1) Intraocular portion. This begins at the optic disc or papilla which represents the site of congregation of the axons of the retinal ganglion cells before the fibres leave the eyeball. The diameter of the optic disc is about 1·5 mm. There is usually a slight depression in the optic disc called the physiological cup and through which the central retinal vessels pass. The nerve fibres leave the eyeball through the openings of the lamina cribrosa (which is a sieve-like area in the posterior sclera).

(2) Orbital portion. The nerve fibres from the eye become medullated as they enter this portion outside the lamina cribrosa. From there, they run a slightly curved course to the optic canal being enclosed by meninges. The central retinal artery pierces the meninges about 11 mm behind the eyeballs and then enters the substance of the nerve.

(3) The intracanalicular portion lies within the optic canal of the sphenoid bone. The optic canal is narrow and here the nerve accompanied by the ophthalmic artery is particularly liable to damage e.g. fracture.

(4) The intracranial portion extends from the optic canal and the optic chiasma.

CONGENITAL ABNORMALITIES

Coloboma

A defect or hole may be present in the optic disc and this depression varies greatly in size from one patient to another. The coloboma may only be an accentuation of the physiological cup but in some there is an inferior crescentic coloboma along the lower border of the disc (Fuchs' coloboma). When the coloboma is larger the appearance resembles that of glaucomatous cupping.

INJURIES

The optic nerve is prone to be damaged in fractures of the sphenoid bone involving the optic canal. Rarely is the nerve injured as a result of a penetrating injury but an ischaemic necrosis may occur after interference to the blood supply or after pressure from oedema.

After injury to the nerve fibres, they degenerate but the optic disc looks healthy for some days because the degeneration has not yet reached the optic disc. In the case of fracture of the optic canal, optic atrophy is not manifest for 14–21 days.

When damage to the nerve is slight, function may return to normal in a few days but a more extensive injury leaves a permanent scotoma and avulsion results in blindness. The prognosis is poor in the absence of an early return of function.

INFLAMMATION OF THE OPTIC NERVE (OPTIC NEURITIS)

The term applied to inflammation of the optic nerve is optic neuritis. If the inflammation is anterior to the central retinal vessels then changes appear at the optic disc. If the inflammation is posterior to these vessels, the optic disc is then likely to be normal although it may well be atrophic at a later date. Optic neuritis behind the eyeball is referred to as retrobulbar neuritis.

The vision is usually suddenly and dramatically reduced; in severe cases only perception of light is present (rarely a total absence). The visual defect varies greatly from case to case and depends on the extent of damage to the nerve fibres. The direct pupillary responses to light are sluggish while consensual reactions are unchanged. The pupil on the affected side is often moderately dilated.

Rarely the optic disc is normal in the acute phase but usually it is oedematous (particularly with neuritis close to the eyeball). The oedema of the disc is slight and extends only slightly onto the adjacent retina which may also contain some fine haemorrhages.

Sometimes movement of the eyeball on the affected side evokes pain because of pressure of the contracting muscle on the inflamed nerve. Enlargement of the blind spot or a sectorial scotoma may be demonstrated.

In many cases the condition gradually subsides and vision may or may not improve. Atrophy of the optic nerve is usual while the disc margins are hazy.

Optic neuritis may occur in different conditions:

(1) Disseminated sclerosis. About 30% of patients with this disease have retrobulbar neuritis in one or other eye as a presenting feature. The neuritis gradually resolves and seldom is neuritis coincident in the other eye which may be involved at a later date. Apart from pupillary changes, nystagmus may also be present.

(2) Neuromyelitis optica (Devic's disease). Bilateral optic neuritis usually occurs in young people suffering from this disease. Marked atrophy of both optic discs is the rule but recovery of vision after the acute attack subsides varies a lot.

(3) Hereditary optic neuritis (Leber's disease). This condition presents in the late teens or soon afterwards with the rapid onset of bilateral impaired vision. The optic discs become pale and vision remains defective in most, but there is evidence that some improvement occurs with the administration of large doses of Neocytamen.

(4) Optic neuritis is occasionally seen in some of the exanthemata e.g. measles, whooping cough, etc.

Treatment

The course of retrobulbar neuritis may be favourably influenced by systemic steroids or A.C.T.H.

PAPILLOEDEMA

Papilloedema is the name utilised to indicate an oedema of the optic disc. The oedema occurs in a wide variety of circumstances, it may be unilateral or bilateral and it is usually compatible with good vision.

In the early stages the condition may be symptom free, and even when the optic disc is markedly oedematous vision is usually good. Sometimes the oedema extends onto the neighbouring retina to involve the macula; only then will vision fail appreciably. The oedema is accompanied in most cases by small haemorrhages on or near the optic disc. The retinal veins are engorged and tortuous.

The visual fields show enlargement of the blind spot in the early stages but if optic atrophy follows the papilloedema, there is concentric constriction of the visual fields. Other field defects may also be present depending on the causal factors.

Unless the oedema is relieved, the optic nerve becomes atrophic and vision depressed.

Treatment is that of the cause. The causes of papilloedema are varied and numerous. These include: intracranial tumour or space-occupying lesion, severe meningitis, extensive intracranial haemorrhage, raised intracranial pressure (or benign intracranial hypertension), hydrocephalus, uveitis, malignant hypertension, some blood dyscrasias, collagen diseases, orbital lesions obstructing venous return from the central retinal vein, etc.

OPTIC ATROPHY

It is traditional to describe or recognise optic atrophy as being (1) Primary or (2) Secondary.

(1) Primary Optic Atrophy

This atrophy results from disease directly affecting the optic nerve fibrils or from degeneration of the ganglion cells of the retina (whose axons or fibres form the optic nerve fibres) or from trauma. Trauma may cause optic atrophy and here the extent and distribution of the atrophy varies with the extent of the severance of the nerve fibres.

As already mentioned, optic atrophy commonly follows optic neuritis but many cases of syphilis develop an optic atrophy, particularly in the tertiary stage of tabes dorsalis and general paralysis of the insane.

Vascular occlusion of the nutrient optic vessels causes optic atrophy. Nutrient vessels to the ganglion cells of the retina may be occluded and give rise to optic atrophy.

Neoplasms of the optic nerve frequently cause optic atrophy but they will be described presently.

Degenerations of the ganglion cells of the retina are characteristically accompanied by some optic atrophy, while advanced disease of the retina e.g. extensive choroido-retinitis, is eventually accompanied by optic atrophy.

(2) Secondary Optic Atrophy

This form of optic atrophy usually follows pressure on the optic nerve indirectly as a result of a disease process adjacent to the nerve.

This, therefore, is liable to occur in:

(a) pressure on the optic nerve at the optic disc as for example in glaucoma
(b) pressure in the orbit as in orbital cellulitis, orbital tumour, pseudotumour, thyrotrophic exophthalmos
(c) pressure in the optic canal as in fracture of bone, Paget's disease of bone, osseous maldevelopments, sphenoidal ridge meningioma
(d) pressure on the optic chiasma, e.g. pituitary adenoma, aneurysm, arachnoiditis
(e) pressure on the optic tract as in brain tumour.

TUMOURS OF THE OPTIC NERVE

(1) Glioma

This is the commonest neoplasm of childhood which arises from the neuroglia of the optic nerve. The neoplasm is usually unilateral and, as it grows forwards and backwards, gives enlargement of the optic canal. Apart from the demonstrable increase in size of the optic foramen on X-ray visualisation, there is also visual failure and optic atrophy while proptosis is a late manifestation.

(2) Meningioma

This tumour presents in adult life when its slow growth is noteworthy.

The late onset of visual failure and papilloedema are common while proptosis and disordered ocular motility also occur. The tumour arises from the arachnoid sheath of the nerve and does not invade the nerve fibres.

Treatment

Removal of the optic nerve in a glioma is probably desirable. In some cases exposure of the affected area may be easily obtained through a lateral orbitotomy (Kronlein's operation) or by transfrontal orbitotomy.

11 *DISEASES OF THE LACRIMAL SYSTEM*

ANATOMY

The lacrimal gland secretes tears into the outer part of the upper fornix of the conjunctiva. The tubulo-racemose lacrimal gland is situated in the upper and outer part of the orbit just posterior to the orbital margin. The gland is about the size of an almond and its secretory nerve arises from the facial nerve, passing to the gland via the greater superficial petrosal nerve.

The tears formed in the lacrimal gland pass into the conjunctival fornix and across the front of the cornea towards the lacus lacrimalis of the conjunctiva. From there tears pass into the adjacent lacrimal puncta: one punctum is on each lid near the medial ends.

Each punctum is the external opening for the lacrimal canaliculus of that lid. Each canaliculus passes vertically into the lid from the punctum before coursing horizontally and medially for about 7 mm to enter the lacrimal sac near its upper end. Frequently, the canaliculus from the upper lid and that from the lower lid join together to form the common canaliculus which joins the lacrimal sac.

The lacrimal sac lies in the lacrimal fossa which is delimited by the anterior and posterior lacrimal crests. The vertically placed sac is about 12 mm long with its blind upper end (fundus) just above the medial palpebral ligament. The lower part of the sac joins the nasolacrimal duct.

The nasolacrimal duct passes downwards and slightly outwards and backwards in close contact with the maxillary antrum to open into the inferior meatus of the nose. Drainage of tears is largely dependent upon an effective pumping action by the orbicularis oculi muscle.

LACRIMATION AND EPIPHORA

Excessive watering may be due (1) to an over-production of tears (lacrimation) in the presence of patent tear passages or (2) to inadequate drainage of the tears (epiphora).

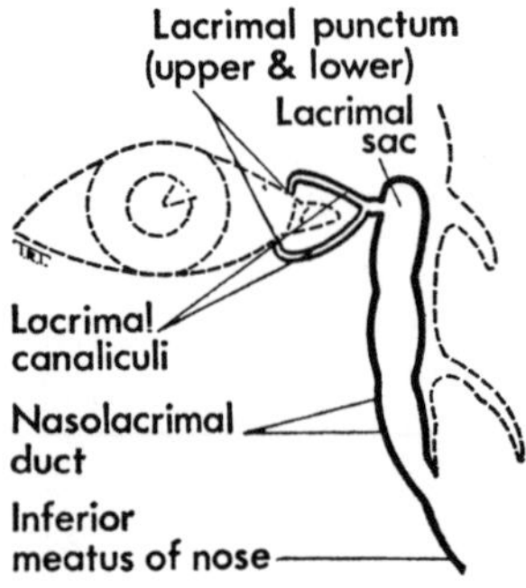

FIG 17 Diagrammatic representation of passages for drainage of tears

Lacrimation

Lacrimation is caused by some emotional stimuli. In addition, it may follow irritation or inflammation of the conjunctiva, cornea and anterior uvea. Raised intraocular tension, as in acute congestive glaucoma and exposure to bright light, can also produce lacrimation. Treatment is directed to the removal of the provoking cause.

Epiphora

Malapposition of the lacrimal punctum or stenosis of the punctum will produce epiphora. Occasionally, epiphora is caused by impaction of a lash or foreign body in the punctum. In others obstruction of the canaliculus prevents adequate drainage of tears so that epiphora arises. Infection in the canaliculus is uncommon but when present may be due to the fungus actinomycosis. The canaliculus may be severed as a result of trauma; should this happen, early plastic repair of the canaliculus is desirable before the torn canaliculus becomes embedded in fibrous tissue. The insertion of a polythene tube into the torn canaliculus forms a rigid structure around which the lacerated lid tissues may be repaired.

Obstruction at the junction of the lower end of the sac and the upper end of the nasolacrimal duct gives rise to epiphora. Tears accumulate in the lacrimal sac, which then passively dilates to become distended with mucus and sometimes pus (mucocoele). This mucopus may be expressed upwards via the puncta by pressing on the skin overlying the mucocoele.

Stagnation of tears within the lacrimal sac causes infection and this also quickly involves the sac wall—dacryocystitis. The inflammation is acute or chronic.

Dacryocystitis is commonly of sudden onset and a tender swelling of the sac pushes up the injected overlying skin. Occasionally, pointing of the contained pus occurs and in the absence of response to systemic antibiotics release of the pus affords relief. Fortunately the improvement from systemic antibiotics is dramatic.

A chronic dacryocystitis is associated not only with a shrunken lacrimal sac but also with a chronic conjunctivitis. Treatment of a mucocoele is by dacryocystorhinostomy (union of the sac lumen with that of the nose) or by dacryocystectomy in the elderly.

Tumours of the lacrimal sac are a rare cause of epiphora.

Obstruction of the nasolacrimal duct is sometimes associated with inflammation or neoplastic change in the maxillary antrum.

Congenital obstruction of the nasolacrimal duct is seen not infrequently in the newborn. Here, canalisation of the duct is delayed for several weeks after birth so that the features of conjunctivitis with mucopurulent discharge from the punctum is justifiably treated by local antibiotic. Should the obstruction persist until 3–4 months of age, probing and syringing of the affected lacrimal passages are usually effective in relieving the epiphora and infection—a lacrimal probe is passed into the punctum along the lacrimal passages into the inferior meatus of the nose. A light general anaesthetic is required for this manoeuvre.

Epiphora is commonly present with paresis of the orbicularis oculi muscle (e.g. facial paresis or Bell's palsy) because of ineffective pumping of tears along the passages by the weakened muscle fibres surrounding the canaliculi and sac.

Impaired Tear Secretion

Reduced tear formation is most commonly associated with disease in the lacrimal gland e.g. neoplasm, inflammation, atrophy or damage to the secretory fibres (trigeminal nerve) of the gland. Tears may, however, be normally produced but not be passed to the conjunctiva because of a blockage of the channels by disease. One of the more common atrophic conditions of the gland is known as Sjogren's Disease.

Tumours of the Lacrimal Gland

These are rare and tend to be of two main types,(a) the adenoma or 'mixed-cell tumour' and (b) the adenocarcinoma.

The slowly growing firm tumour presents as a mass in the upper outer part of the orbit during middle age. As the mass enlarges, the eye becomes pushed forwards (proptosis) and downwards while the ocular movements are limited and tear secretions diminished. Once the diagnosis is established excision of the tumour is often effective but radiotherapy may also be utilised.

12 *DISEASES OF THE ORBIT*

ANATOMY

The roof, floor, medial and lateral walls constitute the bony limits of the orbit. All four walls tend to converge posteriorly to the apex of the orbit while the walls terminate anteriorly at the orbital margin.

There are three main apertures in the orbit:

(1) The Superior Orbital Fissure, which is a space formed between the greater and lesser wings of the sphenoid bone. This fissure is an important route of communication between the middle cranial fossa and the orbit for the transmission of the 3rd, 4th and 6th cranial nerves, branches (lacrimal, frontal and nasociliary) of the ophthalmic division of the 5th cranial nerve, the superior and inferior ophthalmic veins and various recurrent arterioles and sympathetic nerve filaments.

(2) The Inferior Orbital Fissure is the space formed between the greater wing of the sphenoid bone, the orbital process of the palatine bone and the maxilla. The fissure transmits the infraorbital artery, branches from the inferior ophthalmic vein to the pterygoid plexus, branches of the maxillary division of the 5th cranial nerve, and secretory fibres to the lacrimal gland.

(3) The Optic Canal is formed by the two roots of the lesser wing of the sphenoid and connects the middle cranial fossa with the apex of the orbit. The canal transmits the optic nerve surrounded by the pia, arachnoid and dura maters of the meninges, cerebrospinal fluid and the ophthalmic artery.

The extrinsic ocular muscles have been described in connection with strabismus. The connective tissue of the orbit forms fascial condensations which will be mentioned where necessary, while the orbital fat is one of the major constituents of the orbit.

CONGENITAL ABNORMALITIES

A maldevelopment in the formation of the bones of the skull during earlier intra-uterine life wherein premature union of one or more of the sutures occurs is referred to as dysostosis. This premature union sometimes impairs development of the brain.

(1) Oxycephaly or tower skull is a vertical elongation of the skull due to premature synostosis. Papilloedema may be observed in the early stages but most cases are seen after the synostosis has been present for some time and the papilloedema has been replaced by optic atrophy. The orbits are shallow and the eyes prominent (proptosis) while divergent strabismus is usual.

(2) Hypertelorism

In this condition, there is premature ossification in the sphenoid bone and an excessive separation of the eyes is obvious. The wide interpupillary distance (even 20 or

30 mm in excess of the normal interpupillary distance of about 60 mm) gives the face a 'bovine' look. A divergent strabismus is usual.

(3) Scaphocephaly is the name given to an antero-posterior elongation of the head with transverse narrowing.

Intermediate variants of the above anomalies occur while asymmetry in the orbits is also seen. For example, a small orbit develops in the presence of a small eye (microphthalmos) and a large orbit may be present with a large eye as in buphthalmos.

(4) Meningocoele

A defect in the orbital wall permits protrusion of a pouch of meninges containing cerebrospinal fluid into the orbit from the cranium. The defect is usual between the frontal and ethmoid bones. Although the defect is commonly unilateral, it may be bilateral and the pouch may be large enough to contain cerebral tissue (meningo-encephalocoele).

(5) Dermoid Cyst

This inclusion cyst usually presents in the upper and outer part of the orbit but it is sometimes also found towards the upper and inner part of the orbit. The cyst occasionally becomes inflamed and contains a variety of tissues. An intraorbital dermoid causes proptosis. Gradual enlargement of a dermoid cyst is the rule. Treatment is excision once the cyst is large enough to justify removal.

INJURY

Orbital Haemorrhage

Orbital haemorrhage may result from severe contusion. Ecchymosis (haemorrhage into the tissues) and subconjunctival haemorrhage are the rule, while proptosis occurs with larger haemorrhages. Absorption of the haemorrhage is usual. Occasionally, orbital haemorrhage follows a penetrating injury to the orbit.

Fracture

Fracture of the orbital bones may occur without bony displacement and leave little or no residual defect. On the other hand, fracture with bony displacement can cause widespread disorders. For example, such a displacement involving the floor of the orbit allows not only an herniation of the orbital contents into the maxillary antrum but may also permit infection from the antrum to invade the orbit. It is therefore desirable to endeavour to reduce the fracture and particularly to free any of the extrinsic muscles of the eye which are caught in the fracture.

INFLAMMATION

Orbital Cellulitis

This acute inflammation of the orbit may arise from a variety of conditions. The infection may be introduced with a penetrating injury of the orbit or spread from an adjacent infected nasal sinus. Occasionally, infection reaches the orbit via the blood stream i.e. the organisms being transported in the blood from some other distant focus of infection.

In orbital cellulitis there is marked injection (redness) and oedema of the lids and conjunctiva while pain accompanies ocular movement and is followed by restriction of ocular movement. As the orbital oedema increases there is proptosis and congestion of the retinal veins while in the more severe cases there is even strangulation of the blood supply to the optic nerve. Raised temperature and pulse are common during the acute phase.

TREATMENT

Adequate and early systemic antibiotic therapy offers the most effective relief. Rarely, nowadays, is drainage of any abscess formation needed.

Cavernous Sinus Thrombosis

In this condition, infection spreads to the sinus and precipitates clotting of the blood in the cavernous sinus. Infection enters the cavernous sinus directly or from another focus of infection (usually in the face, orbit or nasal sinuses).

The conjunctiva becomes congested and the globe proptosed while ocular movements become more and more impaired because of involvement of the 3rd, 4th and 6th cranial nerves coursing forwards in the sinus to supply the extrinsic ocular muscles. In addition, the 3rd cranial nerve involvement causes paralysis of accommodation and the pupil to be fixed and dilated because of paresis of its pupillary fibres. The 5th cranial nerve becomes paralysed in the cavernous sinus and causes anaesthesia of the cornea. The stagnation of blood in the involved sinus impairs venous return from the eye and causes papilloedema. Because of venous communications between the right and left cavernous sinuses the clinical features tend to be bilateral.

Early and energetic systemic antibiotic therapy is essential.

Pseudotumour of the Orbit

There is some evidence suggesting that this condition is secondary to orbital infection but it is also found in conjunction with a medley of apparently dissociated conditions. Pathologically, there appears to be necrosis of orbital fat. The fat cells become infiltrated by round cells and the cells are replaced by fibrous tissue. As the fat necrosis increases so does the amount of fibrous tissue.

The clinical findings are similar to those of orbital tumour hence the term pseudotumour. Oedema and injection of the lids and conjunctiva are usual while impaired ocular movements are manifest. Pain is common but irregular in onset, nature and duration. Proptosis tends to progress and may become so marked that it hazards the cornea by exposing it (the lids do not close adequately across the proptosed eye). Papilloedema is present in some but optic atrophy appears in others because of strangulation of the blood supply to the optic nerve by the fibrous tissue. Spontaneous arrest eventually occurs but this is seldom seen before advanced orbital fibrosis has caused marked disruption in the orbit. Systemic steroids and antibiotics besides orbital irradiation have been of much therapeutic value.

EXOPHTHALMOS DUE TO THYROID DYSFUNCTION

Exophthalmos is a common manifestation of thyroid disorder.

Thyrotoxicosis

In this condition, there is excessive production of thyroxine (thyroid hormone). Clinically, upper lid retraction and exophthalmos are early features. The upper lid tends to lag behind the cornea on downward movement of the eye. The ocular muscles become weak and inadequate convergence appears.

Thyrotrophic Exophthalmos

This arises during the course of thyrotoxicosis and is believed to arise from excessive production of thyrotrophic hormone by the basophil cells of the anterior pituitary.

Exophthalmos and ophthalmoplegia characterise the condition in which orbital oedema is predominant. The lids and conjunctiva are oedematous while the upper lid develops a mechanical retraction which prevents adequate lid closure. This causes an exposure keratitis and in untreated cases leads to hypopyon ulceration and panophthalmitis. Oedema of the extrinsic ocular muscles results in their disordered function. Optic atrophy and visual field defects have also been reported.

The main aim of treatment is to rectify the endocrine disorders but the safety of the cornea is an early consideration and tarsorrhaphy is desirable before exophthalmos becomes too marked. Some protection is given to the cornea by antibiotic administration particularly in oculentum form. When the exophthalmos is marked, orbital decompression is desirable to protect the eyes. This may be by the transfrontal approach or via the lateral wall of the orbit. Once the condition has become stabilised, surgery to the extrinsic ocular musclature may relieve diplopia.

TUMOURS OF THE ORBIT

Tumours may arise in the orbit itself when they are known as primary ones or they originate outside the orbit and spread into it—secondary tumour.

(1) Primary

Haemangioma

This is one of the commoner orbital tumours usually appearing in childhood and presenting with proptosis. The proptosis increases with crying or straining and may even be pulsatile but otherwise causes little upset. The typical haemangioma is often small and does not require treatment although irradiation may produce a decrease in size.

Reticuloses

This is the term applied to several tumours of the haemopoietic system and comprised of lymphoma, lymphadenoma, lymphosarcoma and reticulosarcoma. They may present as a soft palpable mass in the orbit which may cause proptosis. Often they occur in scattered foci and surgical excision is therefore difficult or impossible so irradiation or cytotoxic drugs may be employed.

Sarcoma

This malignant tumour is typically found in children. The embryonal sarcoma or rhabdomyosarcoma arises in the extrinsic ocular musculature and causes chemosis and injection of the conjunctiva. As it increases in size, proptosis is more evident and the irregular vascular fleshy mass may become palpable. Treatment is seldom permanently effective and surgery (in the form of exenteration) or irradiation achieves a transient improvement.

Other tumours may also be primary in the orbit e.g. lacrimal gland tumours, osteoma, neurofibroma, etc., but they will not be described here.

(2) Secondary

These are usually carcinomata from the nasal sinuses and nasopharynx but may be a secondary carcinoma from breast, prostate and bronchus. However, a meningioma or glioma can also spread into the orbit from the cranial cavity. Extraocular spread of a uveal malignant melanoma or a retinoblastoma to the orbit is also seen.

13 *GLAUCOMA*

ANATOMY

Glaucoma is the term applied to the presence of raised intraocular pressure (above the normal level).

The intraocular pressure is largely dependent upon the structures within the eyeball but especially upon the vitreous and the aqueous humour. The volume of vitreous tends to alter within minor limits except in exceptional circumstances (e.g., following vitreous loss after trauma). The aqueous, on the other hand, varies according to (1) the rate of its production by the ciliary body and (2) the rate of its filtration (or removal) through the filtration spaces at the angle of the anterior chamber.

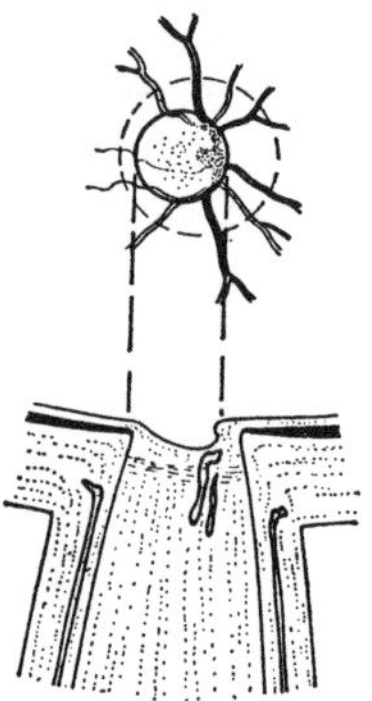
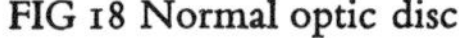

FIG 18 Normal optic disc

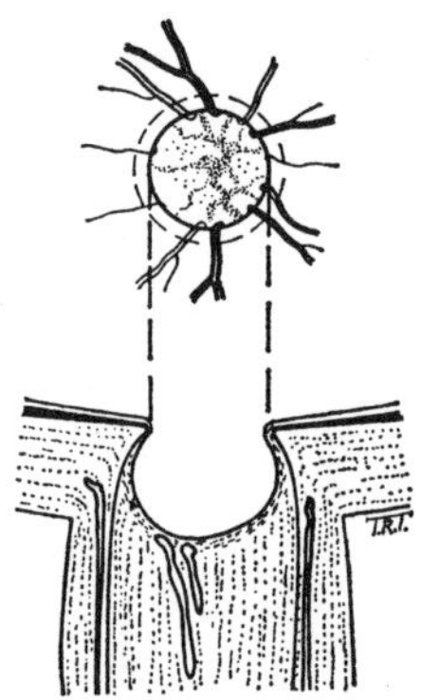

FIG 19 Glaucomatous optic disc

The intraocular pressure varies during 24 hours (diurnal variation) and tends to be highest in the morning. The range of normal intraocular pressure is between 18–25 mm Hg, as recorded with a Schiötz type of tonometer, and slightly less with an applanation tonometer.

The intraocular tension may be roughly assessed by digital tonometry. This entails an assessment of the pressure required to indent the downward looking eye with the forefinger placed on the upper lid.

A more accurate method of estimating intraocular pressure is by using a tonometer. The cornea is anaesthetised and the tonometer is placed on the cornea. The central plunger of the tonometer indents the cornea and the tonometer scale reading is noted. This is then translated into mm Hg. The reading is fairly accurate.

A more precise estimate of the intraocular pressure is obtained by the applanation tonometer which measures the pressure required to flatten a small portion of the cornea.

Tonography

In tonography, a tonometer is applied to the cornea for about four minutes and the change in intraocular tension during this time is measured. From a knowledge of the initial intraocular pressure and the pressure after four minutes it is possible to determine the coefficient of the facility of outflow (C). The normal eye has an outflow coefficiency of more than 0·14 while an impaired outflow is usually indicated by a value lower than 0·12. That is, when the value of C is less than this figure, an impediment to the outflow of aqueous from the eye is present.

PRIMARY GLAUCOMA

(1) Infantile Glaucoma (Buphthalmos)

This form of juvenile glaucoma has been recognised for many centuries, largely because of the gross enlargement of the eyeball caused by raised intraocular pressure. There is maldevelopment at the filtration angle of the anterior chamber where mesodermal remnants persist and impede the outflow of aqueous, usually in both eyes.

Due to increased intraocular pressure, there is a progressive enlargement of the globe and an increase in the diameter of the cornea which may well remain clear for a long period. Eventually, splits in Descemet's membrane and oedema appear in the cornea to cause its opacification. The anterior chamber is deep and the optic disc becomes cupped and atrophic. The enlarged eye is myopic and photophobic. If the intraocular pressure remains high, the eye becomes blind.

TREATMENT

Rarely is it possible to maintain the intraocular level at a satisfactory level by miotics. Surgery offers the most effective form of relief and here, goniotomy is most lasting. A goniotomy knife is introduced into the anterior chamber and the mesodermal remnants at the filtration angle of the chamber are incised under direct view.

(2) Chronic Simple Glaucoma (Open-angle Glaucoma)

The cause of the raised intraocular tension in this condition seems to lie in changes in the trabeculae of the filtration spaces. There is an obstruction to the outflow of aqueous. Characteristically, the disease presents after the age of 40, although a few cases occur in the young.

In the early stages, this glaucoma exhibits few if any symptoms. Seldom does the patient experience any pain or ache in the eye, and only occasionally does he complain of impaired vision in the early stages.

Examination of the eyes characteristically shows no loss in visual acuity until the condition is advanced. On the other hand, a good visual acuity is compatible with appreciable field loss which is demonstrable on charting of the fields. With the perimeter, the early field loss is typically in the nasal quadrants, but the loss spreads towards fixation point and, once it is reached, the visual acuity is irreparably diminished. Charting of the central fields on the Bjerrum screen shows field loss much earlier. The periphery of the field shows diminution peripheral to the blind spot (Fig. 20). As the loss continues, the blind spot may be gradually isolated (i.e. till it is 'bared') outside the periphery of the now constricted field of vision. Furthermore, a scotoma (area of defective vision) may then appear within the field of

90
0
30
25
20
15
10
5
5
10
15
20
25
30
180
Test Objects
====10/2000 White
2/2000 White
270

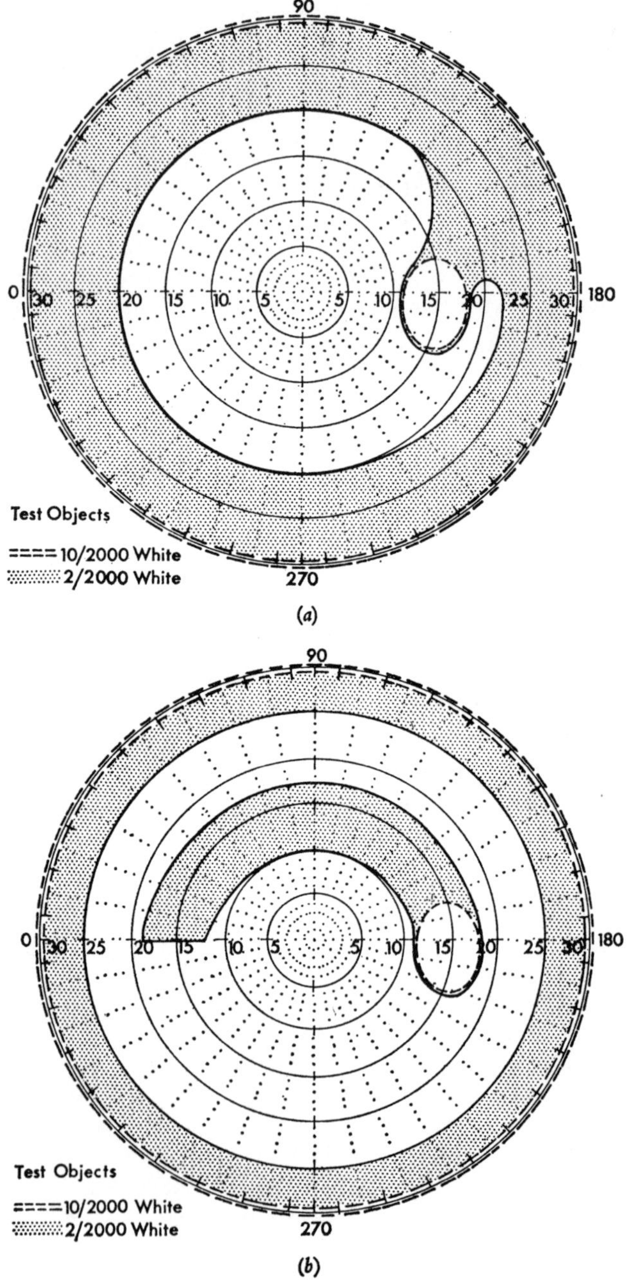

(*a*)

(*b*)

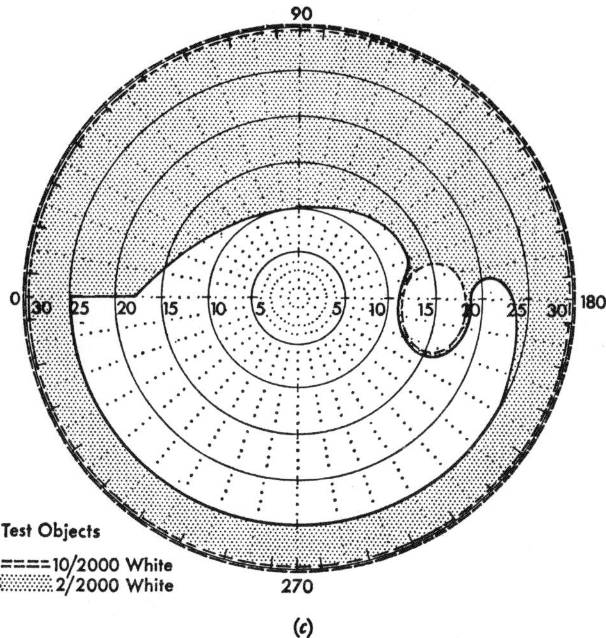

(*c*)

FIG 20 Central field changes in glaucoma (scotoma is shaded area)

vision, arching from the blind spot above and below fixation—an arcuate scotoma. As the loss continues, the field diminishes towards the centre till only a small island of central vision is present before even it is finally extinguished, resulting in blindness. The intraocular tension is raised in most patients. Generally, the pressure varies during 24 hours (i.e. diurnal variation) but in glaucomatous patients the maximum tension recorded is even higher. In some doubtful cases of glaucoma, it is desirable to record the ocular tension during the day at four hourly intervals i.e. phasing so that an abnormal isolated elevation may not escape notice.

In glaucoma the raised intraocular tension causes the optic nerve fibres to degenerate. These fibres atrophy and the optic disc is not only atrophic or pale but the optic cup within the disc also grows larger till it extends to the disc margin—glaucomatous cupping.

It is possible to visualise the filtration angle of the anterior chamber with a gonioscope. Gonioscopy of the filtration angle in chronic simple glaucoma shows the angle to be open.

Tonography reveals a diminished facility of outflow. The facility (C) is less than 0.13 while the ratio of the initial tension (Po) recorded on tonography and the facility i.e. Po/C is greater than 100 (in non-glaucomatous subjects this ratio is less than 100).

The water drinking test is a provocative test for chronic simple glaucoma. The test is easily conducted in early morning when the patient avoids breakfast and any fluid intake before the onset of the test. The ocular tension is noted and the patient asked to drink one litre of water within 5 minutes. The ocular tension is recorded at 15 minute intervals during the succeeding 1½–2 hours. Normal subjects exhibit little or no rise in intraocular tension during the test but glaucomatous patients characteristically show a rise in tension of more than 4 mm Hg.

Treatment

The local application of drugs has been in force for many years. These drugs are varied and numerous.

One group is the anticholinesterase drugs. They inhibit anticholinesterase which normally destroys acetylcholine at the myoneural junctions. These drugs cause miosis, are applied to the eye in drop form and include the following:

eserine ¼% or ½%, rarely 1%
D.F.P. (di-isopropyl fluoro-phosphonate) 0.025% or 0.125%
phospholine iodide 0.06% to 0.25%
The last two are strong drugs liable to irritate the eyes.

Pilocarpine used as drops in concentrations of 1–4% also lowers the intraocular tension and acts directly on the muscle fibres causing miosis. This drug not only diminishes aqueous secretion but also reduces the aqueous outflow resistance at the filtration angle.

Another drug which acts like pilocarpine but *without* having any miotic action is laevoepinephrine. It is only of value in open angle glaucoma and is contraindicated in the presence of a narrow filtration angle.

Intraocular tension can also be reduced by the oral administration of carbonic anhydrase inhibitors, such as acetazolamide (Diamox) 250 mg three times a day or dichlorphenamide (Daranide) 50 mg three times a day. These drugs inhibit the secretion of aqueous by the ciliary body. Diamox also occasionally causes paraesthesiae and renal colic but is otherwise without side effects. Another drug which may be administered orally to reduce intraocular tension is glycerol but it can only be used for short periods.

The intravenous administration of urea and mannitol lowers the intraocular pressure but this intravenous therapy can only be maintained for short periods.

The surgical treatment of chronic simple glaucoma aims in most operations to secure adequate drainage of aqueous from within the eye through a surgically fashioned channel outside the eye to the subconjunctival tissues. In trephine anterior sclerectomy and anterior flap sclerotomy operations, the opening is made near the limbus with a peripheral iridectomy adjacent to the drainage opening. Sometimes, one or more pillars of iris are fashioned and project through the sclerotomy (iris inclusion) to facilitate aqueous drainage to the subconjunctival tissues.

Another type of operation is cyclodialysis, where a track is made to enable aqueous to drain from the anterior chamber into the suprachoroidal space. This operation is of value in aphakia.

A further measure which surgically reduces the intraocular tension is cyclodiathermy (surface or penetrating). Diathermy is applied to the ciliary body and causes a hyaline degeneration which decreases secretion of aqueous. Rarely is cyclodiathermy used as an initial procedure but rather for advanced glaucoma in which other measures have failed.

(3) Closed-angle Glaucoma (Acute or Congestive Glaucoma)

As the name suggests the filtration angle is narrowed and closed by irido-corneal contact. The iris may be pushed forward from behind (as in pupillary block when aqueous does not circulate through the pupil but builds up pressure in the posterior chamber) on to the cornea. When the pupil of an eye with a narrow angle dilates, the iris gathers in the angle and may occlude the filtration spaces. Both these circumstances produce contact between the iris and cornea at the angle of the anterior chamber where the irido-corneal contact (peripheral anterior synechiae) impedes the outflow of aqueous through the filtration spaces there.

In the subacute phase the raised intraocular tension causes aching, some blurred vision or haloes round lights. These features are transient and become more prolonged as the condition passes into the acute or congestive phase. The eye of congestive glaucoma is red, watering excessively (lacrimating), painful while the vision is markedly impaired.

An acute attack is dramatically sudden in its onset with the eye markedly injected. The cornea is hazy because of corneal oedema while the anterior chamber is shallow, the iris oedematous and the oval pupil is dilated. The pupillary reactions to light are impaired and absent in severe glaucoma. Usually it is not possible to see the optic disc during an attack of acute congestive glaucoma because of the corneal oedema. However, in the early stages the optic disc appears healthy and only in the advanced stages does any glaucomatous cupping of the optic disc appear. Likewise, visual field changes are late features. When it is possible to view the angle of the anterior chamber, gonioscopy reveals the angle to be narrow and even closed by peripheral anterior synechiae. The intraocular tension is markedly raised.

In the prodromal phase before the onset of an acute attack, it is possible to do provocative tests to determine the probability of an acute attack ensuing. These are dependent on the fact that pupillary dilatation gathers the iris towards its root where it is bunched up and may occlude the filtration spaces of the narrow angle. This then causes a marked rise of tension. Mydriasis may be achieved by confining the person in a dark room (usually for an hour in this test) or by the topical application of a weak mydriatic e.g. homatropine 1%.

Treatment

A subacute closed-angled glaucoma often responds to repeated guttae eserine ½% or pilocarpine 2%. Some cases, however, continue to maintain raised intraocular tension and become an acute attack. An acute attack demands the early instillation of oily eserine 1% every five minutes for 15 minutes, thereafter every 15 minutes to the affected eye. At the same time, it is desirable to instil guttae eserine 1% once or twice to the fellow eye to obviate the onset of an acute attack in it. A further aid to the reduction of intraocular tension is the administration of 250–500 mg acetazolamide at the same time as intensive miotic therapy is commenced. Many patients vomit during an acute attack so it is preferable to give acetazolamide intramuscularly or intravenously. Alternatives to this drug are intravenous urea, mannitol and glycerol. Failing a satisfactory reduction in tension to around or within normal limits, after 6–8 hours it is desirable to resort to surgery.

Surgical relief of the acute attack involves opening the anterior chamber through a limbal incision and performing either a peripheral or broad iridectomy or including a pillar of iris in the incision (i.e. iris inclusion); the choice of operation largely lies with the surgeon. In many cases of closed-angle glaucoma a prophylactic peripheral iridectomy is done to prevent an acute attack. Before doing this prophylactic surgery, it is desirable to ascertain that the facility of outflow, C, as determined by tonography is above 0.13. If C is less than this, peripheral iridectomy alone will not likely suffice.

SECONDARY GLAUCOMA

Secondary glaucoma occurs as a complication of or in conjunction with a wide variety of conditions. Some of these will be listed below and briefly discussed.

1. The presence of occlusion of the pupil following severe uveitis obstructs the forward flow of aqueous through the pupil (the iris is bowed forwards—iris bombé). Pupillary block may also arise when vitreous herniates forwards, as in aphakia, or when the lens is congenitally misshapen.

2. The anterior chamber may not reform quickly after a glaucoma or cataract operation. As a result iris adheres to the trabeculae of the filtration angle thereby preventing the drainage of aqueous. Loss of the anterior chamber also follows penetrating wounds and aqueous may leak from the wound leaving a shallow anterior chamber and irido-corneal contact.

3. Peripheral anterior synechiae (P.A.S.) formed as a result of forward displacement of the iris as in dislocation of the lens or with some neoplasms of the anterior uvea.

4. The filtration angle may be blocked by organisation of debris deposited there e.g. inflammatory P.A.S.

5. Neovascularisation of the anterior surface of the iris (rubeosis iridis) notably occurs in thrombosis of the central retinal vein, long standing retinal detachment and diabetic retinopathy. The new vessels pass between the iris and the filtration spaces of the angle obstructing them and thereby causing the tension to rise.

6. The filtration angle may become obstructed by the deposition of 'debris'. For example, in a large hyphaema, the angle becomes packed by numerous blood cells which occlude or block the filtration spaces and thereby raise the intraocular tension. Similarly, the deposition of inflammatory cells from an anterior uveitis and debris from pseudo-exfoliation of the lens capsule in the angle can cause the

tension to rise. Sometimes, an extra-capsular cataract extraction or penetrating injury of the lens may cause liberated lens matter to enter the aqueous and become deposited in the filtration spaces. Following cataract extraction it is usual for vitreous to prolapse forwards through the pupil towards the cornea as its support from the lens has been removed. When the vitreous is fluid, it passes to the filtration spaces which then become clogged by vitreous and the hindrance to aqueous outflow causes the intraocular tension to rise.

Treatment

It is initially desirable to treat the cause of the glaucoma as early treatment of the underlying cause may prevent a rise in tension. For example, a severe uveitis should be treated with a mydriatic and steroids. However, once glaucoma is established, the tension may be reduced by oral acetazolamide 250 mg once to three times a day together with treatment of the cause. Some cases do not even respond to these measures and one must resort to surgery—with each case the indications for a particular operation vary.

14 *STRABISMUS*

ANATOMY

There are six extrinsic ocular muscles which move each eye: four recti muscles and two oblique muscles.

The four recti muscles (medial, inferior, lateral and superior) arise from a tendinous ring called the annulus of Zinn which surrounds the optic foramen at the apex of the orbit. From their origins, they course anteriorly around the optic nerve towards the sclera into which they are inserted by flattened tendons situated about 5–8 mm from the limbus.

The superior oblique muscle arises from the bony apex of the orbit above the optic foramen and runs forwards close to the roof and medial walls of the orbit to reach the trochlea or pulley of the superior oblique muscle. The muscle passes through this pulley before continuing laterally below the superior rectus muscle to be inserted into the upper and outer part of the posterior sclera.

The inferior oblique muscle arises from the maxilla (lateral to the orbital opening for the nasolacrimal duct). The fleshy muscle passes laterally and below the inferior rectus muscle to be inserted into the outer and lower posterior sclera.

The lateral rectus muscle is supplied by the 6th (abducens) cranial nerve and the superior oblique muscle is innervated by the 4th (trochlear) cranial nerve while the remaining muscles are supplied by the 3rd (oculomotor) cranial nerve.

ACTIONS OF THE MUSCLES

MUSCLE	ACTIONS
Lateral rectus	Abduction
Medial rectus	Adduction
Superior rectus	Elevation Adduction Intorsion
Inferior rectus	Depression Adduction Extorsion
Superior oblique	Depression Abduction Intorsion
Inferior oblique	Elevation Abduction Extorsion

DEVELOPMENT OF NORMAL BINOCULAR VISION

In normal binocular vision, the two eyes are used together and the development of this depends on:

1. Normal anatomical conditions i.e. normal reflex pathways: ability of an image to be formed on the retina; ability of the stimulus to be transmitted along the visual pathways to the brain; ability of the motor impulse to be transmitted to the extraocular muscles.
2. Awareness and attention. This development occurs by means of the binocular reflexes and these are conditioned and depend upon vision and reward gained (except for the first one which is unconditioned and is postural).

The binocular reflexes evolve so that each new reflex is built up on the previous one, and each must be to some extent established before the next can develop.

Binocular vision is not innate and present at birth. It has to be built up as a child grows, like the use of a limb.

Two fundamental factors must be present:

1. Ability to appreciate with each eye separately an image which must be comparable in each eye.
2. Ability to fuse the two separate images in the cortex.

The ability to appreciate an image with each eye separately depends upon:

(a) Visual acuity value of the retinal receptors.
(b) Ability to hold the eyes in correct alignment to enable bifoveal fixation to take place. This process involves both anatomical and physiological factors.

Once the binocular reflexes are fully developed, they are established for life. They are said to have reached unconditioned fixity by the age of seven or eight years.

Binocular vision (the use of both eyes at the same time) is divided into three grades:

1. *Simultaneous Perception*

The ability to appreciate two different images, one falling on each retina, but not necessarily to superimpose them.

2. *Fusion*

The ability to appreciate two similar images, one falling on each retina, and to mentally blend them and see them as one.

3. *Stereopsis*

The ability to fuse two similar images, one in each eye, falling on slightly disparate retinal elements, and to appreciate them as a single image with depth.

Each grade of binocular vision is said to be built upon the previous one. Therefore, simultaneous perception may exist alone, but fusion cannot be present without simultaneous perception, and stereoscopic vision cannot exist without both simultaneous perception and fusion.

If binocular vision develops normally, with time and correct usage during the first few years of life, binocular single vision will be established. This is the ability to use the two eyes together simultaneously in order to perceive a single image. The process involved is the mental fusing of the two images received by the retinae. These images are slightly dissimilar, and because of this a fine appreciation of depth results with a more accurate judgement of distance in everyday life. This is the reward for binocular single vision, which will encourage good visual acuity in each eye and also parallelism of the visual axes with a good cosmetic appearance.

The degree of development of binocular vision at the time of onset of a squint, determines the prognosis and type of treatment. The longer normal development is allowed to continue the stronger will be the fusion faculty and the easier it will be to repair binocular single vision.

PROJECTION AND NORMAL FIXATION

Light from an object enters the eye and forms an image on the retina. The retina is made up of a series of minute 'receiving cells'—the rods and cones. The cones are responsible for acute and detailed vision; and the fovea, or point of clearest vision, is made up exclusively of cones. The fovea is the point used for fixation, and when one wants to look at an object the eye is moved so that the image falls on the fovea. A line drawn from an object of fixation through the nodal point to the fovea is known as the visual axis.

An image formed on the fovea is always interpreted as being straight-ahead i.e. is projected back along the visual axis.

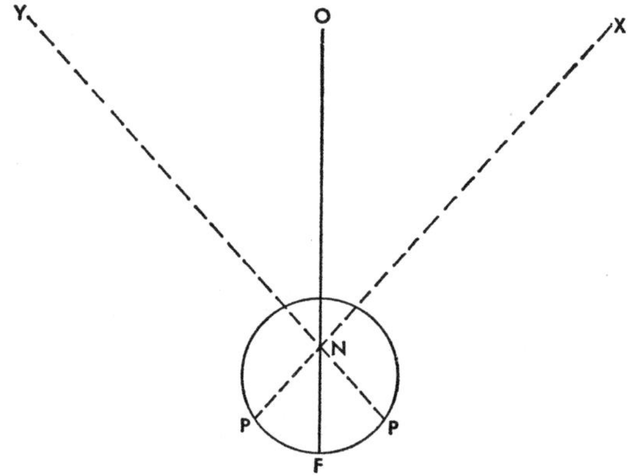

FIG 21 O—Fixation object
N—Nodal point (a theoretical point just behind the pupillary aperture, through which all light rays pass when entering the eye)
F—Fovea
OF—Visual axis

Similarly, all retinal points have a definite visual direction or projection. All those on the left of F will project to the right of O, and vice versa.

Both eyes fix on an object so that an image is formed on each fovea. Both are interpreted as being straight-ahead and they are then mentally blended so that the observer interprets the two images as one object.

Since the two foveae have the same visual projection they are known as corresponding points. The whole of the two retinae are built up of a series of corresponding points, and every retinal element in one eye has a corresponding retinal element in the other eye. Each pair have the same visual projection and are the same distance in the same direction, from the foveae.

Normally, both eyes are used together so that the two foveae receive images of the fixation object. This normal condition is binocular single vision.

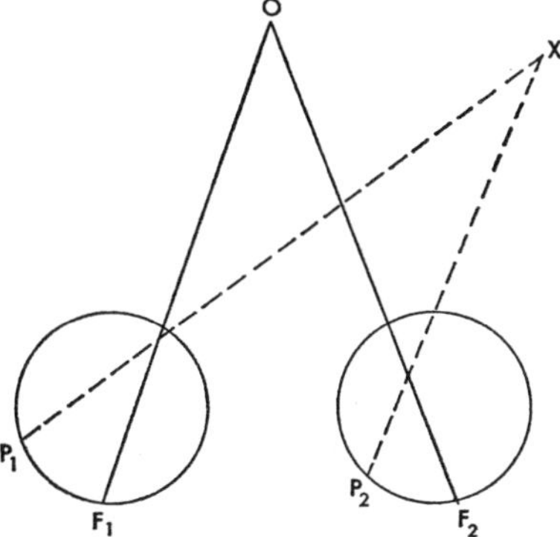

FIG 22 Normal retinal correspondence

AETIOLOGY OF SQUINT

The development of binocular vision may be impeded or prevented and a squint may result. All squints are due to one or more obstacles occurring during the development of the binocular reflexes.

I Sensory

(a) *External obstacles*

(1) Dim illumination—may cause spasmus nutans in infants.
(2) Prolonged uniocular activity—due to incorrect spectacles, using one eye the whole time, prolonged occlusion, ptosis.

(b) *Dioptric obstacles*

Obstacles which interfere with the correct formation of images on the retina.

(1) Errors of refraction.
(2) Opacities in the media
e.g. Ophthalmia neonatorum
Corneal opacities
Injuries or keratitis
Congenital cataract
Heterochromic cyclitis
Retrolental fibroplasia.

(c) *Retino-neural obstacles*

Any lesions of retina or optic nerve. Retarded development or myelination in the visual tract. Toxoplasmosis.

(d) *Proprioceptive obstacles*

(1) Defective ocular proprioception.
(2) Defective non-ocular proprioception.

Impulses arising from muscle are conveyed to C.N.S. and thus we can correctly n tate ourselves and judge the relative position of objects.

II Motor

Cranio-facial dysostosis, oxycephaly, hypertelorism.

(a) *Abnormalities of orbits and adnexae*

This may cause deviation of the visual axis of one eye without an apparent displacement of eyeball due to:

(1) Lesion of orbit or adjacent structures such as a tumour.
(2) Congenital abnormalities in shape or position of orbit.
(3) Injury either to orbit or adjacent structures. These may give appearance of a palsy (relative) but there is no damage to the muscles so there is not a real palsy.

(b) *Condition affecting muscle itself*

(1) Aplasia or abnormal muscle insertion.
(2) Injury to the muscle.
(3) Contracture of antagonist of paralysed muscle.
(4) Disease of the muscle, progressive muscular dystrophy.

(c) *Conditions affecting nerves*

(1) Injury to the nerve.
(2) Inflammation and infection, as in middle ear disease with the 6th cranial nerve affected—Gradenigo's syndrome.
(3) Vascular disease.
(4) Growth, tumour, etc., causing pressure.

(d) *Conditions affecting nerve roots and nuclei*

(e) *Supranuclear lesions*

Paralysis of conjugate muscle movement.
(Note: Eyes may work normally together.)

(f) *Decompensation of ocular muscle imbalance*

(g) *Convergence insufficiency*

III Central

So called because these objects are all related to higher centres of the brain.

(a) *Physical or mental trauma*

(1) Jealousy } etc.
(2) Anger }

These cannot cause a constant squint unless there is already a latent squint.

(b) *General hyper or hypo excitability of C.N.S.*

(1) Teething.
(2) Lethargic state.

(c) *Central uniocular inhibition*

Retinal rivalry, probably not enough by itself but one of many factors causing child to squint.

(d) *Inability of child to learn*

Pathological deficiency in co-ordination of motor ability.

The slightest obstacle in a young child may cause a squint, whereas in an adult or older child when the reflexes are more stable and to some extent developed, a squint will not occur so easily. It may take a series of incidents to cause a squint.

The younger the child, the easier it is for a squint to occur, because the reflexes are not, or hardly, developed and vice versa.

SQUINT (STRABISMUS)

A squint or strabismus is a condition in which binocular single vision is no longer maintained. One eye fixes on the fixation object and the other eye deviates. The deviation may occur in any direction and may be:

LATENT (HETEROPHORIA)—when the deviation is controlled by fusion and is therefore only apparent on dissociation of the two eyes.

MANIFEST (HETEROTROPIA)—when the deviation is present the whole time.

ESOTROPIA/PHORIA OR CONVERGENT SQUINT—when one visual axis deviates inwards.

EXOTROPIA/PHORIA OR DIVERGENT SQUINT—when one visual axis deviates outwards.

HYPERTROPIA/PHORIA (ELEVATION)—when one visual axis deviates upwards.

HYPOTROPIA/PHORIA (DEPRESSION)—when one visual axis deviates downwards.

CYCLOTROPIA/PHORIA—when the vertical meridian of one eye is rotated inwards or outwards (paralytic).

A squint may be:

1. Constant or intermittent deviation.
2. Uniocular or alternating deviation.
3. Concomitant (non-paralytic) or incomitant (paralytic) deviation.
4. Combination of a horizontal and vertical deviation.

CONCOMITANT SQUINT

Esotropia (Convergent Squint)

Tonic

This term is applied to a constant convergent deviation in which the size of the angle of squint remains the same at all distances, with and without glasses.

Accommodative

This term denotes a deviation which is affected by the effort of accommodation, so that the deviation increases for near fixation and without the hypermetropic correction.

There are three types:

1. FULLY ACCOMMODATIVE

Where correction of the refractive error restores binocular single vision i.e. there is no manifest deviation with the glasses.

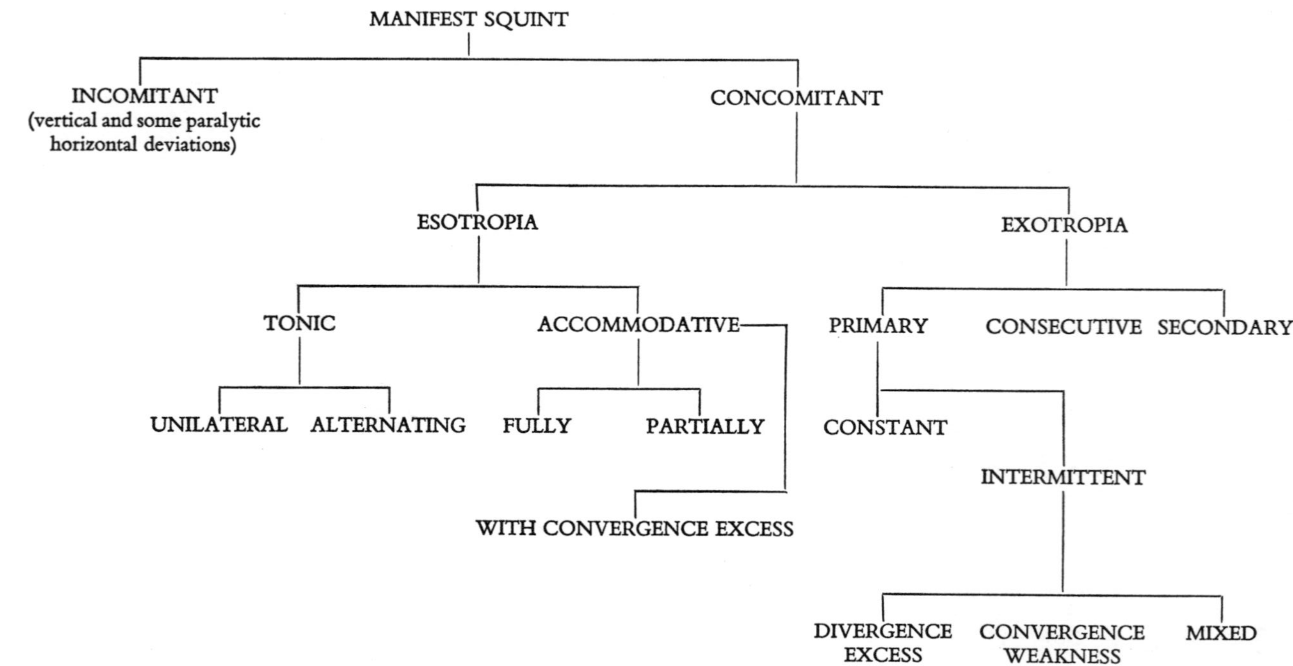
MANIFEST SQUINT
INCOMITANT
(vertical and some paralytic horizontal deviations)
CONCOMITANT
ESOTROPIA
EXOTROPIA
TONIC
ACCOMMODATIVE
PRIMARY
CONSECUTIVE
SECONDARY
UNILATERAL
ALTERNATING
FULLY
PARTIALLY
CONSTANT
INTERMITTENT
WITH CONVERGENCE EXCESS
DIVERGENCE EXCESS
CONVERGENCE WEAKNESS
MIXED

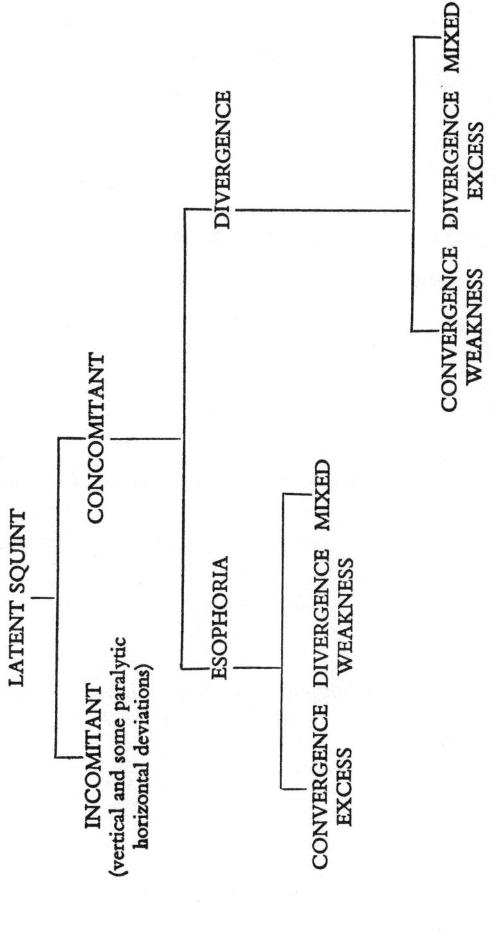
LATENT SQUINT
INCOMITANT
(vertical and some paralytic
horizontal deviations)
CONCOMITANT
ESOPHORIA
DIVERGENCE
CONVERGENCE
EXCESS
DIVERGENCE
WEAKNESS
MIXED
CONVERGENCE
WEAKNESS
DIVERGENCE
EXCESS
MIXED

2. PARTIALLY ACCOMMODATIVE
Where correction of the refractive error reduces the manifest deviation but binocular single vision is not restored.

3. ACCOMMODATIVE SQUINT WITH CONVERGENCE EXCESS
Where the effort of accommodation produces a manifest deviation for near.

Esophoria

This is a latent convergent deviation divided into three types, dependent on which fixation distance the deviation is maximum.

1. CONVERGENCE EXCESS
Where the deviation is greater for near.

2. DIVERGENCE WEAKNESS
Where the deviation is greater for distance.

3. MIXED
Where the deviation is approximately the same for near and distance.

Exotropia (Divergent Squint)

Primary

This primary exotropia may be constant or intermittent, and the intermittent deviation may be divided into three types—dependent on which fixation distance the deviation is maximum.

1. DIVERGENCE EXCESS
Where the deviation is manifest for distance and latent for near.

2. CONVERGENCE WEAKNESS
Where the deviation is manifest for near and latent for distance.

3. MIXED
Where the deviation may be manifest for near or distance.

Consecutive

This term is applied to a divergent deviation which was originally convergent. The cause may be surgery and/or lack of fusion.

Secondary

This term is applied to a divergent deviation generally associated with a blind eye.

Exophoria

This is a latent divergent deviation divided into three types, dependent on which fixation distance the deviation is maximum.

1. DIVERGENCE EXCESS
Where the deviation is greater for distance.

2. CONVERGENCE WEAKNESS
Where the deviation is greater for near.

3. MIXED

Where the deviation is approximately the same for near and distance.

Convergence Insufficiency

This is a common condition which gives rise to symptoms such as eye strain and headaches associated with close work. It is a result of defective convergence and can be easily treated by convergence exercises.

INCOMITANT SQUINT (see paralytic section, page 97)

SIGNIFICANCE OF SQUINT

When a manifest squint occurs i.e. when one eye deviates and binocular single vision is lost, diplopia will be the result.

Diplopia

This is the double vision which occurs when similar images are formed on non-corresponding retinal areas.

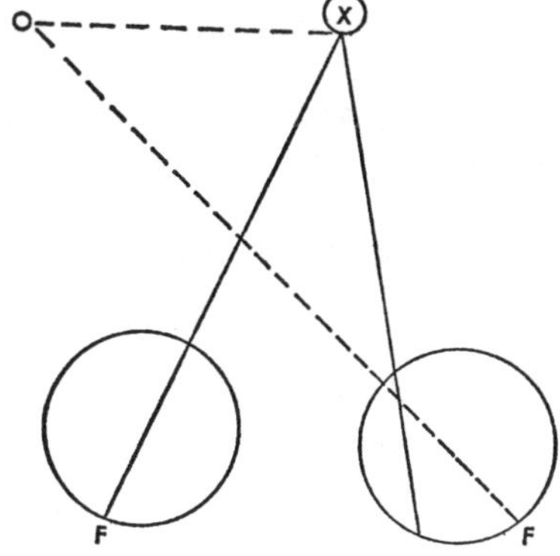

FIG 23 Confusion

Obviously, constant diplopia is intolerable and adaptations are rapidly learnt to overcome this. These may be:

1. *Suppression*

This is the mental inhibition of the image falling on the retina and occurs to restore single vision.

2. *Amblyopia*

This is a deterioration of the visual acuity in the deviating eye, and occurs as a result of prolonged suppression. The younger the child, the more rapidly the amblyopia will develop, and if the condition is not treated quickly the visual acuity may be permanently affected. Treatment should be completed before the end of the developmental period i.e. before the age of eight years.

3. *Abnormal Retinal Correspondence*

This is a condition in which the fovea of the fixing eye is used in conjunction with a point other than the fovea of the deviating eye. This form of retinal correspondence occurs as an adaptation to squint in some cases, and allows a form of binocular vision with fusion and stereopsis.

The presence of any deviation and the resulting adaptations can prevent normal development so that binocular single vision may not be achieved.

PROGNOSIS

The prognosis in any case of squint depends entirely on whether the patient has binocular single vision or the ability to attain it. This means that normal development must have taken place up to the age of at least three years before the onset of squint. This normal binocular vision can be regained with immediate treatment, but can never be developed later in life, thus the age at onset really determines the prognosis.

INVESTIGATION OF CONCOMITANT SQUINT

All patients should have had an eye examination and refraction before attending the Orthoptic clinic.

Investigation in all cases of squint is carried out to assess the visual acuity and state of binocular vision, and to measure the angle of deviation.

1. History

From the history, the age at onset and attributed cause will aid in both the diagnosis and prognosis.

2. Visual Acuity

This should be tested with and without glasses if worn, for near and distance. The vision is tested monocularly with a graded test type, and the presence of any amblyopia will be demonstrated.

3. Cover Test

A simple test used mainly to detect the presence of a manifest squint (heterotropia) or a latent squint (heterophoria) and it forms the basis of the diagnosis.

Method

Seat the patient comfortably with the head straight. Ask the patient to look at a fixation object.

A. *Test for a Manifest Squint (Heterotropia)*

Cover each eye in turn with an occluder while watching the opposite eye. If either eye moves to take up fixation when the other is covered a heterotropia is present. Movement *outwards* means the eye was turned *in*, esotropia—manifest convergence.

Movement *inwards* means eye was turned *out*, exotropia—manifest divergence.

Movement *upwards* means eye was turned *down*, hypotropia—the deviation may be uniocular or alternating.

If neither eye moves to take up fixation then both eyes must be fixing on the object and thus no manifest squint is present. Once this has been established, one can go on and test for the presence of a heterophoria.

B. *Test for a Latent Squint (Heterophoria)*

Cover each eye in turn but this time watch the eye that has been covered as the cover is removed.

If the eye moves *outwards* to take up binocular fixation it has been turned *in*—esophoria.

If the eye moves *inwards* it has been turned *out*—exophoria.

If the eye moves *down* it has been turned *up*—hyperphoria.

If the eye moves *up* it has been turned *down*—hypophoria.

Sometimes the cover must be moved backwards and forwards from one eye to the other to bring about dissociation and make the heterophoria noticeable.

It is very important to note the rate of recovery to binocular single vision when the cover is removed. It may be graded—rapid, moderate, slow, lagging, delayed.

Both with a manifest and latent deviation it is important to note whether the deviation is slight, moderate or marked.

General Points to Remember

1. It is important to use print or a small picture for fixation at near so that accommodation is stimulated and normal reading conditions are more closely reproduced than with a light.

2. The patient's head must be straight and he must be looking straight ahead.

3. If a reading correction is worn, the near cover test must be done with this, with the lower segment of bifocals if these are worn.

Other Information that may be Gained from the Cover Test

1. One has an opportunity to study patient's appearance and may observe:

(a) Cosmetic appearance.
(b) Facial asymmetry.
(c) Epicanthus.
(d) Ptosis.
(e) Abnormal head posture.

2. Position of pupillary reflections may be noted. Eccentric reflection may indicate:

(a) Manifest deviation.
(b) Eccentric fixation.
(c) Angle kappa. This is the angle formed by the visual axis and the mid-pupillary axis.

3. Inability to maintain steady monocular fixation may indicate:

(a) Poor visual acuity if there is indiscriminate wandering.
(b) Nystagmus if movement is regular. This is a continuous and usually involuntary, oscillatory movement of the eyes.

4. *Ocular Movements*

The patient is asked to follow a light as it is moved in all positions of gaze, and any under or over actions of the muscles are noted.

5. *Synoptophore*

This is an optical instrument used for measuring the angle of deviation and assessing the grades of binocular vision i.e. the state of retinal correspondence and the presence of fusion and stereopsis.

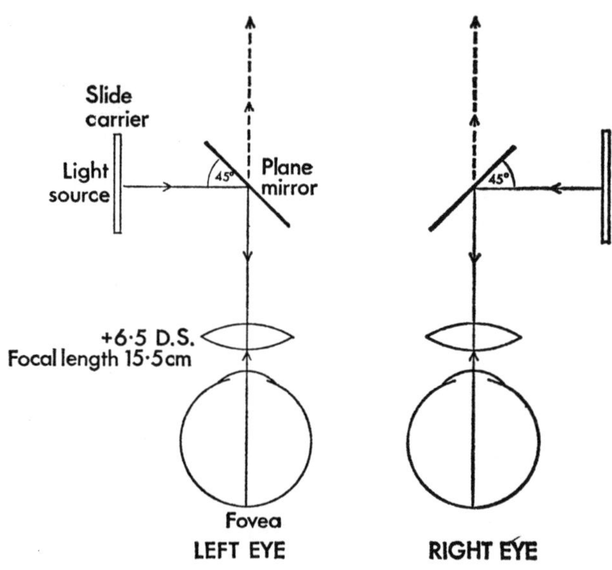

FIG 24 The principle of construction of any major amblyoscope

SIMULTANEOUS PERCEPTION

Dissimilar slides are used such as a lion and cage, and the patient is asked to superimpose the two images. This demonstrates the first grade of binocular vision and the angle of deviation is also registered on a scale marked in degrees and dioptres.

FUSION

Similar slides are used but each picture has a different control. The patient should be able to join the pictures and maintain them joined whilst exercising some convergence.

STEREOPSIS

Similar slides are used which fall on slightly disparate retinal points. The picture should give an appreciation of depth.

6. *Prism Cover Test*

The angle of deviation is measured with and without glasses where worn, for near and distance by means of a prism and the cover test. This accurate measurement is a useful aid in the diagnosis of the type of squint present.

There are various supplementary orthoptic tests which may be used where necessary.

Treatment of any squint consists of one or more of the following:

1. Optical

All patients will have been refracted and the appropriate glasses given where necessary. In most cases, the wearing of glasses affects the angle of squint, and in some cases an increased correction may be given for a time if it maintains binocular single vision.

In accommodative squints, the refractive correction plays a large part in the treatment, especially in fully accommodative squints where the manifest deviation is overcome by the glasses.

Prisms may be used in some cases (generally as a temporary measure) to overcome a manifest deviation or help in the control of a latent squint.

2. Orthoptic Management

Management of Concomitant Squint

Orthoptics is the diagnosis and management of anomalies of binocular vision.

Where treatment of a squint is undertaken the aims are:

(a) To obtain and preserve normal vision in each eye.
(b) To restore comfortable binocular single vision.
(c) To restore a good cosmetic appearance.

A. *Occlusion*

Occlusion is the covering of the good eye to restore normal vision in the amblyopic eye. Most occluders are made of plaster or some form of Sellotape, and the density used depends on the degree of amblyopia present.

Occlusion to restore normal vision is only effective in children up to the age of eight years. After this age, the prognosis for visual restoration is very poor.

Other uses of occlusion:

1. To make the patient more comfortable when diplopia is present.
2. To induce alternation in a uniocular squint.
3. To establish that symptoms are ocular in latent deviations. Binocular single vision is disrupted by occlusion, and hence if the symptoms are eliminated they must be due to the effort of maintaining binocularity.
4. To maintain diplopia pre-operatively.
5. To induce the maximum deviation pre-operatively.
6. To prevent abnormal retinal correspondence in some instances.

B. *Orthoptic Treatment*

MANIFEST SQUINT

The first stage is to overcome suppression and make the patient aware of diplopia when he is squinting. Suppression is overcome by exercises on the synoptophore and also by the use of coloured filters and a light to encourage the appreciation of diplopia.

The second stage is to overcome the deviation if it is only present at times, and is within controllable limits. This may be achieved by the use of glasses and/or drugs and/or orthoptic exercises. Where the deviation is constantly present, or is large, surgery will be necessary.

Exercises to control the deviation involve increasing the range of binocular single vision by fusion of diplopia, and the improvement of fusional convergence. This gives the patient conscious control over the position of his eyes.

Latent Squint

In these cases, symptoms may arise due to the effort of maintaining binocular single vision. Therefore, treatment is aimed at improving fusional convergence to make the control effortless. Where the deviation is large, surgery may be necessary.

Pre- and Post-operative Orthoptic Management

Pre-operatively, patients may be given a short course of orthoptic exercises to overcome suppression and teach awareness of the deviation.

Post-operatively, orthoptic treatment may be given to stabilise binocular vision. Where a residual deviation exists which is within controllable limits, orthoptic treatment and/or drugs and/or clip-on prisms or additional lenses may be used to overcome this. Where the residual deviation is large, more surgery may be needed.

Cosmetic Cases

Where fusion is not present, no attempt is made to obtain binocular single vision. The aim here is to achieve normal vision where possible and a good cosmetic appearance. The orthoptic management merely involves measuring the angle of squint prior to surgery.

3. Drugs

Some miotics, such as D.F.P., and phospholine iodide may be used locally to aid in the control of convergent squint. By producing a peripheral spasm of the ciliary muscle, the effort of accommodation is reduced and therefore the convergence also.

Miotics may be used in suitable cases up to a period of six months, and this form of treatment is generally combined with orthoptic exercises. This method is only successful with patients who have fusion i.e. the potential for binocular single vision, and a small angle of squint.

4. Surgery

Surgical treatment of squint involves the weakening or strengthening of one or more muscles.

Strengthening Operations

RESECTION—muscle shortened and re-attached to insertion.

ADVANCEMENT—muscle severed at insertion and re-attached in front of insertion.

TUCKING—muscle and/or tendon are folded upon themselves and sewn.

WEAKENING OPERATIONS

RECESSION—muscle severed at insertion and re-attached to the globe nearer the origin of the muscle.

PARTIAL MYECTOMY—a portion of the muscle is removed and the ends cauterised.

MARGINAL MYOTOMY—muscle weakened by vertical incisions in the upper and lower borders.

TENOTOMY—tendon of muscle severed completely, and left. For example a typical operation for a convergent squint would be to recess (weaken) the medial rectus and resect (strengthen) the lateral rectus.

A typical operation for a divergent squint would be to resect (strengthen) the medial rectus and recess (weaken) the lateral rectus.

In many cases of squint more than one operation is necessary. The degree of recession or resection carried out depends on the size of the deviation and the condition of the relevant muscles. Most authorities consider a 5 mm recession and an 8–12 mm resection to be the maximum. Although the deviating eye is generally the eye of choice for surgery in the first stage, it does not matter as the defect is binocular.

5. Pleoptics

This is a specialised form of treatment used in some severe cases of amblyopia. Generally in these cases the vision is very low i.e. $< 6/60$ and a condition of eccentric fixation exists and the fovea is no longer used.

The treatment aims at stimulating the fovea to improve visual acuity and restoring normal central fixation.

PARALYTIC SQUINT—INCOMITANT

Paralytic squint must be caused by an obstacle to the motor pathway, that is to say the lesion must affect the muscle, the nerve supplying it, or the nerve nucleus. This condition may be congenital e.g. due to:

(a) developmental anomalies
(b) trauma
(c) disease

or acquired e.g. due to

(a) trauma
(b) general disease
(c) secondary to local disease
(d) general disease affecting muscles
(e) mechanical defects.

A paralytic squint is an incomitant squint i.e. the deviation varies depending on which eye is fixing and on the position of gaze. This incomitance occurs because of the imbalance between the extraocular muscles. The deviation, fixing with the non-affected eye, is known as the primary deviation. The deviation fixing with the affected eye is known as the secondary deviation. The secondary deviation is always greater than the primary due to the increased innervation required to move the affected muscle. Also, the deviation increases when the eyes are turned into the field of action of the affected muscle; and it decreases when looking in the opposite direction.

Investigation

1. *History*

It is important to try to ascertain the cause of the palsy, and the duration.

2. *Diplopia Test*

In a recently acquired condition the patient will have diplopia. The separation of the images will increase as the deviation increases and therefore the greatest separation will be in the field of action of the affected muscle; the false image will be projected into the direction in which the eye cannot move.

3. *Cover Test*

The cover test is carried out in all directions of gaze and will reveal the position in which the deviation is maximum i.e. the field of action of the affected muscle.

4. *Ocular Movements*

Examination of ocular movements in all directions of gaze will generally reveal any abnormalities, i.e. limitations or over-actions.

5. *Synoptophore*

This instrument can be used to measure the deviation in all directions of gaze and fixing with either eye. It will therefore demonstrate the incomitance and position of greatest deviation.

6. *Hess Screen Test*

This is a test used in cases of incomitant squint to plot the movement of each eye. The limitation of movement will be demonstrated by the small field of movement of the affected eye, and particular limitation in the position of the main action of the affected muscle. The larger field of the non-affected eye will demonstrate the excess innervation supplied to the contra-lateral synergic muscles.

ABNORMAL HEAD POSTURES

This is a compensatory mechanism used to move the eyes into such a position that the palsied muscle is not used, and hence the deviation and resulting diplopia are overcome. The position of the head will aid in the diagnosis of the affected muscle e.g. right lateral rectus palsy.

Right Lateral Rectus Palsy

The face will be turned to the right in order to move the eyes away from the field of action of this muscle.

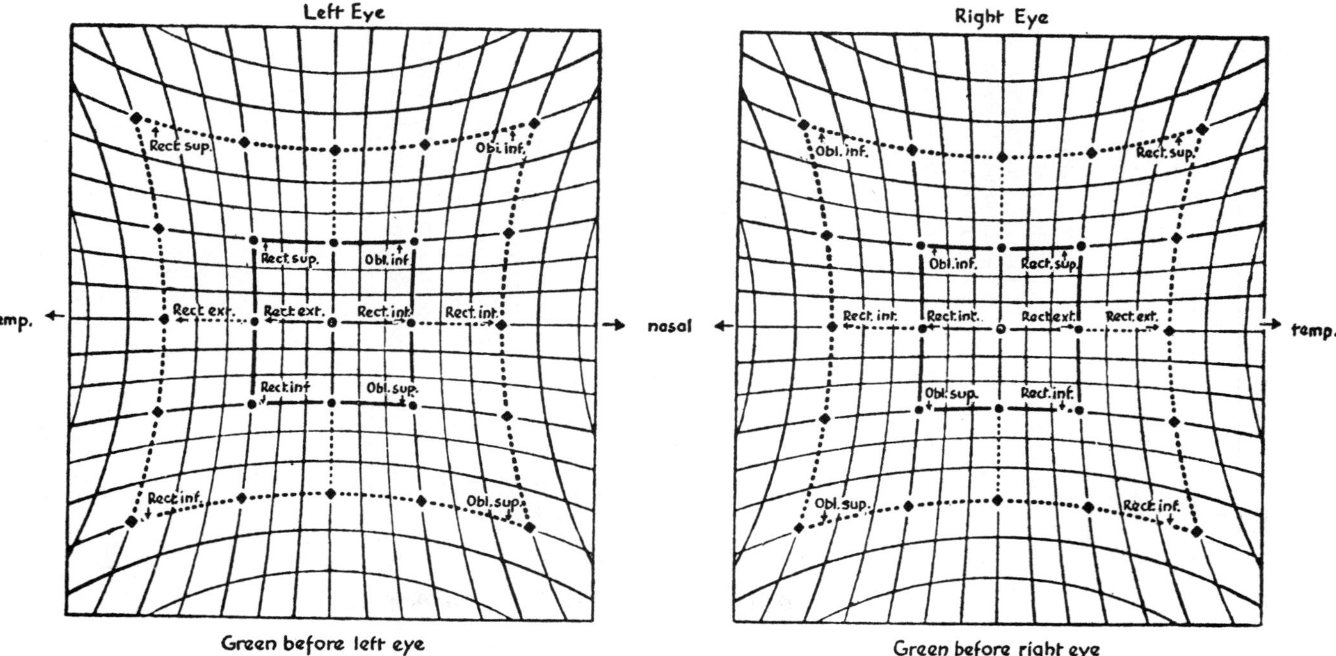

FIG 25 Hess Screen test chart

DIFFERENTIAL DIAGNOSIS OF ACQUIRED AND CONGENITAL OCULAR PALSY

	Acquired	Congenital
Onset	Sudden	Intermittent
Symptoms	c/o diplopia, inability to judge distances, usually distressed by symptoms	If diplopia present patient not as distressed by it. Usually intermittent, occurring when squint becomes manifest.
Abnormal head posture	Always aware of it, to overcome diplopia. No anatomical changes.	Unaware of it, or fails to relate it to his eyes. May have changes in the vertebral column i.e. scoliosis.
Degree of concomitance	Secondary deviation greater than primary i.e. incomitant but degree depends on duration of squint.	Usually concomitant
Suppression	Absent at first, may occur later.	Nearly always present, often amblyopia also.

Importance of Distinction Between Acquired and Congenital

(1) Acquired palsies other than those of traumatic origin may be symptomatic of undiagnosed general disease, such as myasthenia gravis, disseminated sclerosis, etc., which require medical and neurological investigation and treatment.

(2) Acquired palsies may (a) improve (b) deteriorate; in either event treatment is delayed. No surgery is undertaken until at least 6 months after the onset, and only then if condition is static. Congenital palsies are unlikely to change and symptoms are due to decompensation, therefore no need to delay treatment.

(3) Orthoptic *treatment* (as opposed to supervision) may be necessary in cases of *congenital* palsies to *overcome* suppression, whereas in *acquired* palsies the orthoptist should aim to *prevent* suppression in cases unlikely to recover and those which are unsuitable for treatment (e.g. progressive diseases).

(4) Surgical treatment of congenital palsies usually needs to be more extensive because of secondary muscle changes; fibrous attachments, etc., than in cases of *acquired* palsies.

Management

Congenital

1. *Compensated*

Patients in whom some binocular single vision has developed because of an abnormal head posture. If these patients have adequate binocular single vision and are symptom-free no treatment is given. If there is difficulty in maintaining binocular single vision and symptoms result, treatment is given. This is usually surgery and may be combined with orthoptic treatment.

2. *Decompensated*

Patients in whom binocular single vision has not been developed, or cannot be demonstrated.

These patients have a manifest squint but no symptoms as suppression will have occurred to overcome the diplopia. The treatment is surgery in these cases if there is a poor cosmetic appearance.

Acquired

The management depends on the aetiology.

1. *Cases which do not show spontaneous recovery*

These patients are kept under observation for six months or until the condition is static. During this time, an attempt is made to make the patient comfortable by using occlusion, prisms or the teaching of an abnormal head posture to overcome the diplopia.

Once the condition is static, surgery is carried out to overcome the deviation.

2. *Cases which show spontaneous recovery*

These patients are kept under observation and encouraged to maintain their field of binocular single vision by means of an abnormal head posture, prisms or orthoptic treatment.

3. *Cases due to general disease*

These patients are kept under observation to help to determine the cause of the condition. General treatment of the cause is given. Occlusion and prisms are of particular use with these patients to overcome the diplopia.

NYSTAGMUS

Involuntary ocular oscillations characterise the disorder called nystagmus. There are two main groups of nystagmus: (1) Jerk, (2) Pendular.

(1) Jerk

In this form, there is a slow movement in one direction and a rapid movement in the opposite direction to the slow component.

(2) Pendular

The oscillations are equal in speed and amplitude in each direction.

Smaller degrees of nystagmus are easily recognised on viewing the eye with an ophthalmoscope. Nystagmus is generally horizontal but it may be vertical, rotary or even oblique. Seldom is nystagmus restricted to one eye and seldom is it see-saw nystagmus (i.e. one eye turns upwards and the fellow eye turns downwards).

For the sake of classification, three forms, aetiologically distinct, are recognised:

(1) *Ocular Nystagmus*

This nystagmus probably arises because insufficient visual stimuli reflexly maintain normal control of the extrinsic ocular musculature. As a result, there is pendular nystagmus which develops and usually becomes permanent in the newborn or infant up to two years of age.

Several forms are recognised:

(a) Deviational Nystagmus

This occurs in about 50% of normal persons when the eyes are deviated outside the binocular visual field. It is often referred to as nystagmoid jerks.

(b) Optokinetic Nystagmus

This may be evoked once the patient has sufficient vision to perceive the stimulus, be it a rotating drum or a moving light. It is most easily seen by looking at passing objects from a moving train. The nystagmus has a jerky rhythm and is in the direction of the moving stimulus. The reflex is absent in ocular blindness, in lesions of the pathways between the higher visual centres and the frontal motor centre and in lesions of the visual cortex.

(c) Latent Nystagmus

This is an unusual nystagmus seen when one eye is occluded. Typically, the vision in the two eyes is unequal and fine nystagmus is present when the weaker eye is covered. Conversely, coarse nystagmus arises when the stronger eye is occluded.

(d) Amblyopic Nystagmus

This is seen when the normal fixation reflex does not develop because of defective vision. It is observed during the first few months of life and presents in albinism, achromatopsia (colour blindness) besides a variety of congenital abnormalities.

(2) *Vestibular Nystagmus* (*Labyrinthine nystagmus*)

This results from stimulation of the labyrinths. The nystagmus is a jerk nystagmus with fine horizontal and rotatory movements. Clinically, it is found in lesions of the labyrinth or of its subcortical pathways.

(3) *Central Nystagmus*

This is a jerk nystagmus occurring in lesions of any part of the nervous system controlling ocular posture. It is thus present in a wide variety of lesions ranging from vascular, inflammatory, degenerative to neoplastic.

(4) *Congenital Idiopathic Nystagmus*

This nystagmus is of unknown cause and exhibits pendular movements which may become jerky. It is usually present in apparently normal eyes.[1]

15 *NURSING PROCEDURES AND PRACTICE*

BATHING AND SWABBING OF AN EYE

Equipment

5–10 lint squares
1 gallipot
1 jug of normal saline standing in a bowl of warm water

Method

1. Make the patient comfortable with the head supported.
2. Cleanse the unaffected eye first, as this is often slightly encrusted and the patient feels more comfortable as a result; in addition, the patient will then know what to expect when the affected eye is treated and co-operate more readily.
3. The swabs are folded into four, with the fluffy side inwards; the smooth edge and corner are used.
4. The two swabs are moistened in solution and a third dry swab is held between the 3rd and 4th fingers of either hand.
5. The patient is instructed to gently close his eye and the lids are then wiped from the nasal corner outwards; very little pressure is needed. This cleanses the upper lid.
6. The swab is then discarded.
7. The patient is then asked to look up with the eyes open, while the lower lid is cleansed in the same manner with a wet swab; in addition, the loose skin of the lower lid is pulled down to the orbital margin by the thumb of the other hand, thus the cornea is protected from being touched by the swab in the event of nervousness on the part of the patient or nurse.
8. The lower lid generally needs most attention and the number of swabs required varies. The important point is that the eyes must be left clean and all swabs used should be damp but not dripping, care being taken to avoid touching the tip with the fingers.
9. The patient is then asked to close his eyes and the lid margins are dried.
10. This procedure is then carried out upon the affected eye.
11. Often, the upper lid of this eye is encrusted and the patient is asked to 'Close the eyes as if in sleep' i.e. not to squeeze the lids and not to resist the gentle pull on the upper lid in addition to looking downwards.
12. The gentle pull everts the upper lid and, by looking down this time, the cornea is again out of harm's way. *All crusts must be removed* before treatment can be applied effectively.

13. When swabbing eyes following intraocular surgery, great care must be taken to ensure that the swab is not used above the lid margin of the upper lid, as in most instances, the ocular incision is in this area above and is very tender.

INSTILLATION OF DROPS AND OINTMENT

Instillation of Drops

Equipment

Prescribed drops
5 lint squares

Drops are prescribed for many reasons. The great majority contain drugs and therefore must be administered by the nurse *with all the care and precaution she would take when administering drugs orally or by injection*. The dangers of incorrectly administered drops cannot be overstressed. The obvious hazard of a miotic being instilled to one eye and a mydriatic to the other is often quoted, but other less obvious conditions can occur, such as allergy. which can result in great discomfort to the patient.

Method

1. Check the expiry date of the drops on label.
2. Check the drops with the patient's medication sheet for drug percentage, time and eye.
3. Explain the procedure to the patient.
4. Place the patient in a comfortable position with head well supported, especially if intensive treatment is to be carried out.
5. Ask the patient to look up in order to avoid a drop falling directly onto the cornea.
6. Gently pull down and slightly evert the lower lid, instil the drop into the centre of the lower fornix. Unless especially instructed to do so, avoid instilling the drop nasally, as the position of the punctum will cause the drop to be immediately drained into the lacrimal duct. In theory the outer canthus is suggested, but the lower fornix at this point is rather shallow, even when the patient's head is inclined away.
7. Ask the patient to gently close his eyes without squeezing. It is often an advantage to hold down the lower lid for a few seconds after the patient has closed his eye, as this also prevents the drop from being squeezed out. More than one drop can be instilled, but it is considered that two drops are the most the conjunctiva can retain at one time. In certain corneal conditions, and for the removal of corneal sutures, it is necessary for the drops to run directly over the cornea, it must be stressed *to run over*, and *not directly on to*. This can be achieved by asking the patient to look down whilst in a semi-recumbent position, and instilling the drops close to the corneo-scleral

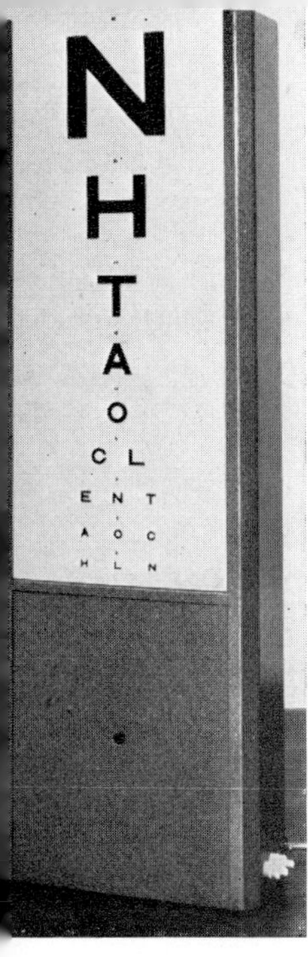

PLATE 8 Distance test-type

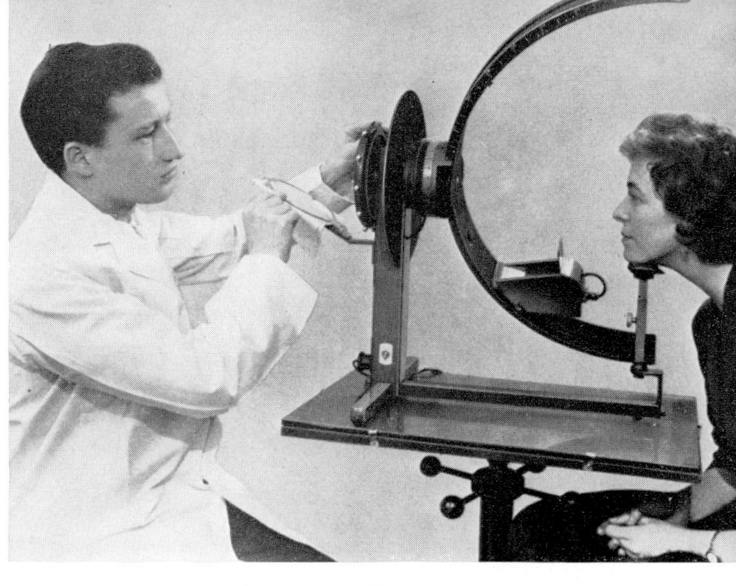

PLATE 9 Recording peripheral visual fields on perimeter

PLATE 10 Requirements for taking a conjunctival culture

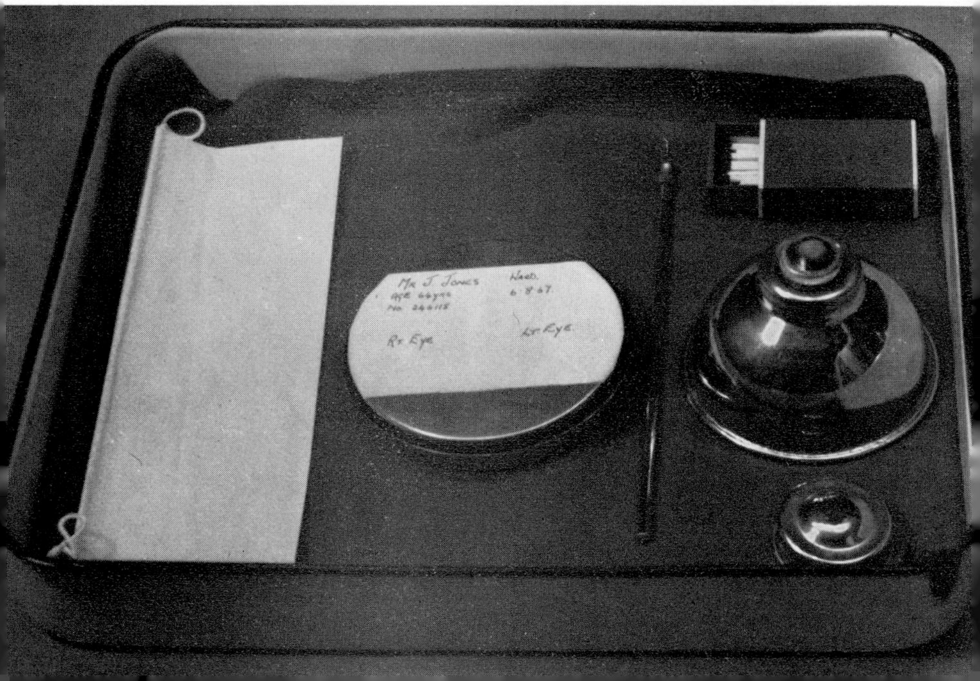

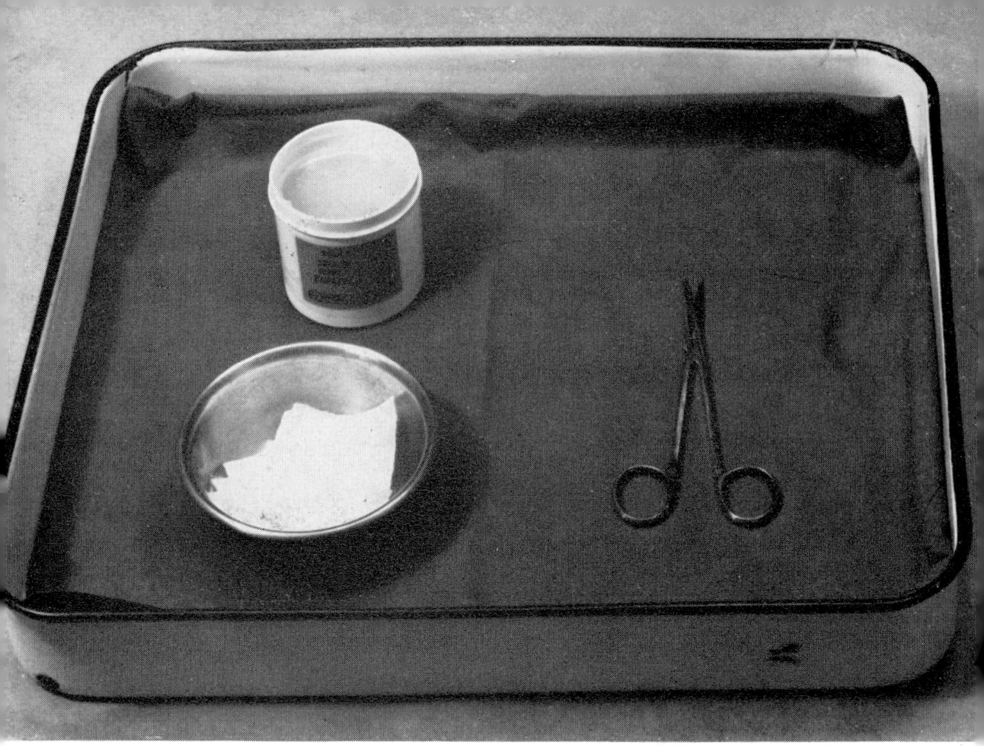

PLATE 11 Equipment for cutting eyelashes

PLATE 12 Apparatus for Schiötz tonometry

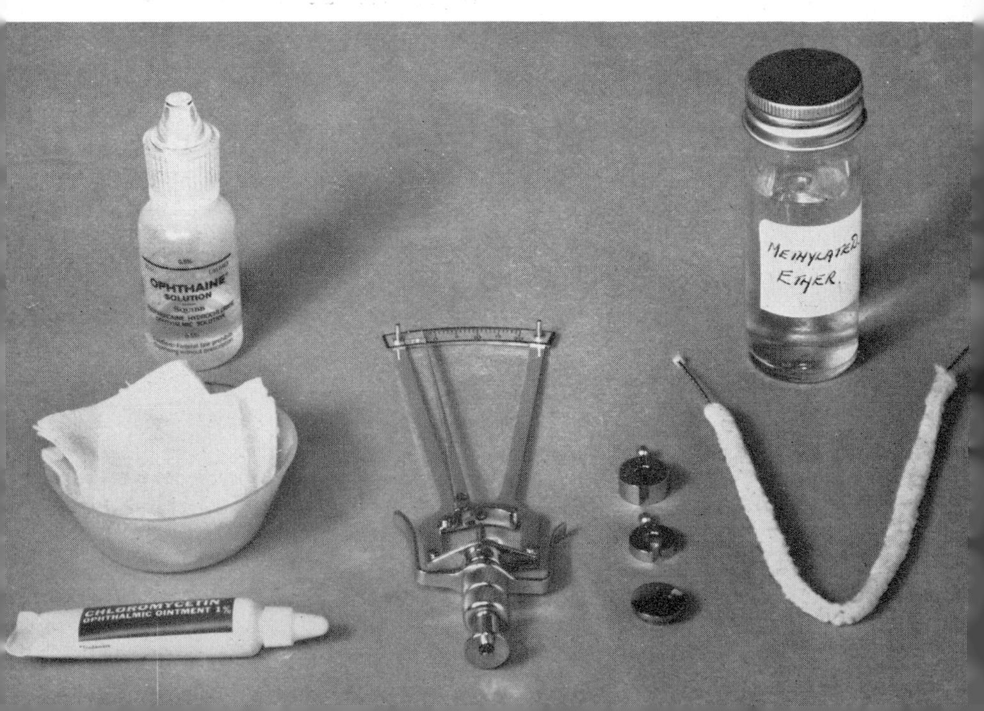

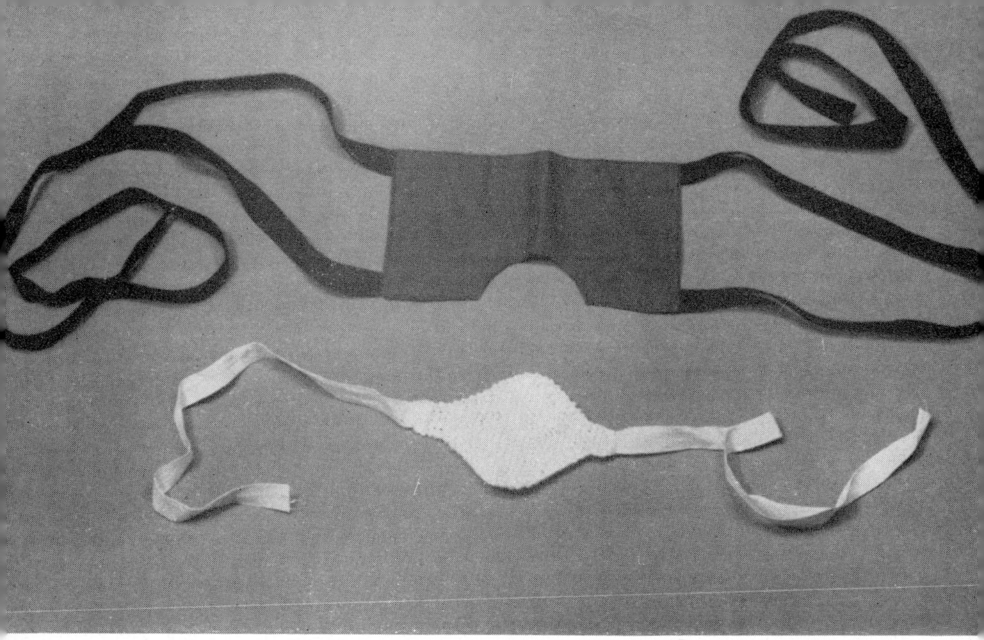

PLATE 13 (top) 'Moorfields' double eye bandage
(bottom) Knitted shade—single eye

PLATE 14 Requirements for syringing lacrimal passages

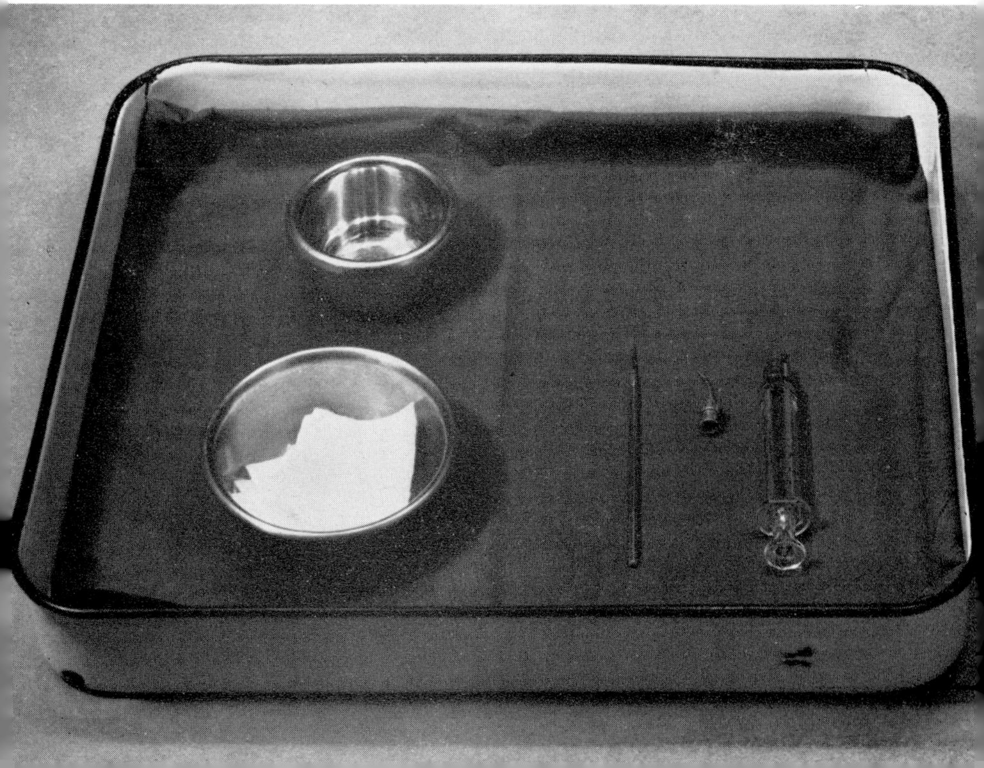

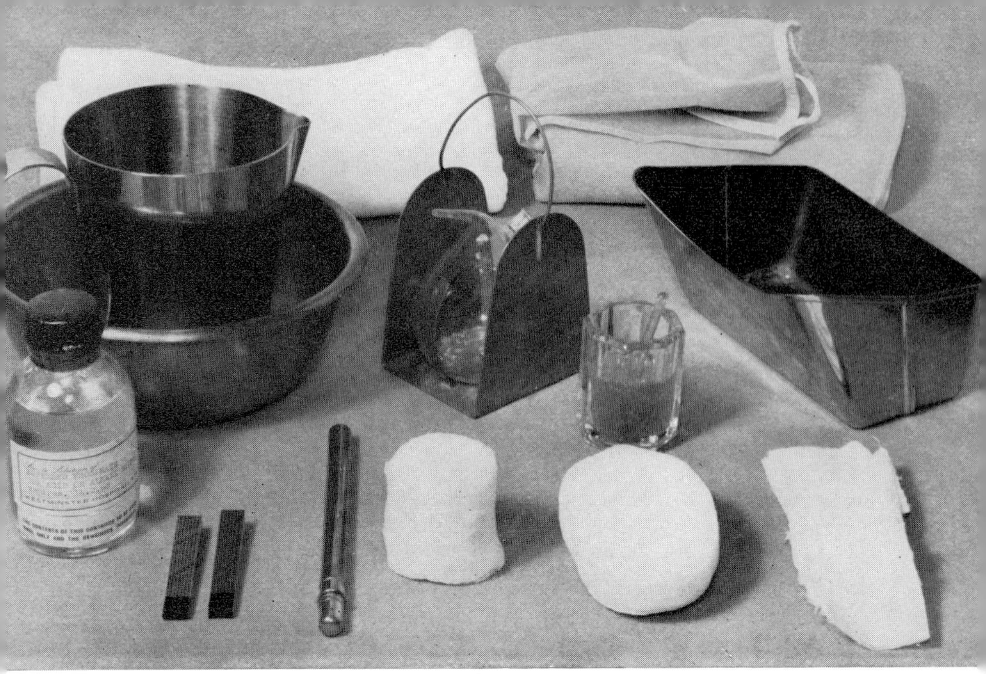

PLATE 15 Equipment for irrigating an eye: (l. to r.) towel, waterproof cape, jug in bowl of warm water, undine in carrier, glass rod in solution, Manchester Dish, buffer solution, litmus paper (red, blue), thermometer, lint squares, eye pads, bandage.

PLATE 16 Requirements for carbolization of a cornea: (l. to r.) guttae, solution of Phenol, bandage, glass gallipot, eye pads, ointment, triangular blotting paper, sharpened orange sticks.

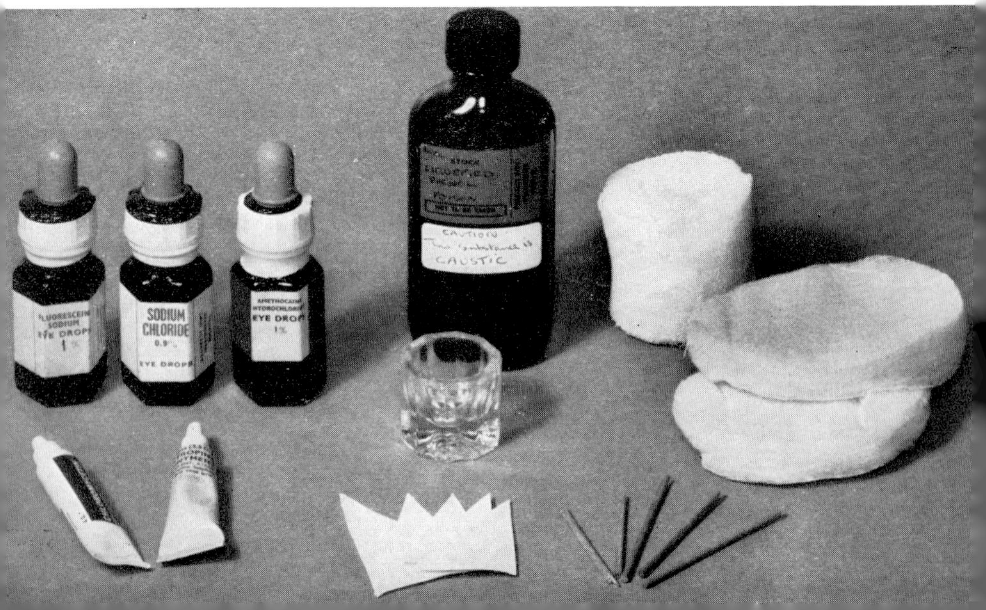

margin superiorly. For local anaesthesia, this method is used after 1 or 2 drops have been placed in the lower fornix.

Instillation of Ointment

Ointment has the advantage that it remains in the conjunctival sac for longer periods, and it is particularly useful at night, as it can be applied on retiring and patients receiving intensive local drops during the day need not be awakened.

The individual tubes of ointment used nowadays make application easier, and of course allow far greater sterility as each patient has his own tube, which is discarded upon his discharge from hospital. The lower lid is slightly everted with a swab, the patient is asked to look up and the ointment is squeezed into the lower fornix, starting at the inner canthus and finishing at the outer canthus. The patient is asked to gently close his eye and any excess ointment is wiped away with the swab.

Application of ointment with a glass rod is still occasionally necessary. The glass rod must be sterile, and closely examined for scratches or chips as these cut and may severely damage the patient's eye. The rounded tip of the rod is dipped into the ointment and the lower lid held down, as before. The patient is asked to look up, the tip of the glass rod is placed in the lower fornix, and the patient asked to gently close his eye, *still looking up*. The glass rod is then gently withdrawn sideways, with a slight twisting movement of the index finger and thumb. Again any excess ointment is wiped away with the swab.

Application of Ointment to Lid Margins

This may be ordered in:

(a) *Conjunctivitis*—to prevent the discharge from drying and sealing the lids together, and to combat infection. The ointment is generally applied at night, the patient being asked to keep his eyes closed during the application. A swab is used to apply the ointment along the lash margin.

(b) *Blepharitis*—to treat this inflammation of the lid margins the ointment should be well rubbed in. Before the application, all crusts must be removed from the lid margins. This is accomplished by patience, perseverance and sodium bicarbonate lotion.

1. The patient is made comfortable with the head supported.
2. The patient is asked to close his eyes and the upper lid is slightly everted by slight pressure on the lid margin.
3. Cotton-wool applicators dipped in sodium bicarbonate lotion are used to remove the scabs, by scrubbing *gently but firmly*.
4. For the lower lid, the patient looks up and the lower lid is drawn down with a lint square.

EYE IRRIGATION

Equipment (Plate 15)

1 undine in metal container
1 glass rod

1 Manchester Dish
10–15 lint squares
2 sterile eye pads
1 jug
1 bowl
1 lotion thermometer
1 mackintosh cape or plastic sheet
1 towel—dressing or paper tissue
1 book of litmus papers
Appropriate solution + guttae Ophthaine 0.5%

If irrigation is to be performed because of caustic substances in the eye, acids, alkalines, etc., litmus paper is used to determine the pH and irrigation performed with the counter irritant, i.e. Acid burn irrigate with alkaline and vice versa. BUT IF THERE IS ANY DOUBT—irrigate with Normal Saline.
Temperature: 38°C (100°F) usually.

All equipment except for a protective cape should be sterile. If not pre-sterilised, the undine should be filled with warm water, placed in a protective stand and then *boiled* in a steriliser.

Method

1. Explain the procedure to the patient.
2. Drape the protective cape and towel around the patient and position the patient. The best position is sitting upright with the head supported by a head-rest, either in a chair or bed, but irrigation can be easily carried out with the patient lying down. In either case, the chin must be horizontal and the head inclined to the side of the eye to be treated. Adequate lighting is essential.
3. Any discharge, ointment or oily drops will have to be first *bathed away*, otherwise difficulty will be experienced in holding the lids apart.
4. Pour correct solution into a jug: the temperature should not be more than 38°C (100°F) unless the prepared solution is to be carried to the bedside, then 40°C (103°F) is needed.
5. The solution is poured over the inside of the nurse's wrist, to make sure that the temperature is comfortable.
6. The patient is then given the Manchester Dish to hold against his cheek, not under the chin.
7. A nurse may stand behind her patient or at the side.
8. The undine should be held in the right hand if the left eye is to be irrigated and vice versa. The reason for this is that the irrigation is commenced nasally and allowed to flow out towards the dish i.e. in a downhill manner. If the undine is held in an incorrect hand the nurse's vision is obstructed. A spare swab is held between the 3rd and 4th fingers until required.
9. The lids are held apart, generally with the 1st and 2nd fingers stretching the loose folds of skin to the orbital margin.

10. Warn the patient that the irrigation is commencing, run some solution over his cheek to make sure that it is comfortable. The undine is held approximately an inch away from the lids:
(a) To prevent contamination.
(b) The higher the undine is held the greater the pressure of the solution; pressure is NOT required, merely a gentle flow.
11. The flow is kept constant once started and is controlled by the index finger over the hole on the spout of the undine. Intermittent trickles are *irritating* to the patient and *inadequate*.
12. The flow is concentrated upon the inner canthus, but the patient is asked to look up, down, to the right and to the left. *Note* The lower fornix must be well irrigated and the upper lid everted, and irrigated especially with caustic burns. *Failure to do either of these* will make the whole irrigation useless.
13. The swab held between the 3rd and 4th finger is used to dry the lids after the irrigation has been completed and only after drying the lids and cheek is the dish removed, otherwise the solution will run down the patient's neck.

Aids to Successful Irrigation

Comfortable position for patient and adequate protection.

Warm solution.

Talk to the patient during the procedure to distract his attention.

Encourage him to keep both eyes open; most adults find that keeping their mouths open makes this easier. Children are often more co-operative if sucking a sweet (a soft one).

If there is severe oedema of the eyelids, they should *never be forced apart* with lid retractors, except upon the surgeon's instructions.

In the case of severe pain, the surgeon will often prescribe guttae Ophthaine 0.5% which is a local anaesthetic drop that does not have the stinging qualities of guttae amethocaine 1%.

TAKING CONJUNCTIVAL CULTURE

Equipment (Plate 10)

1 spirit lamp
1 platinum loop
1 culture plate
1 box of matches
1 mask

This procedure is carried out routinely prior to intraocular operations, and in all cases of conjunctivitis or obvious infection of the eye or lid margins, before any antibiotic therapy is commenced.

Method

1. Explain the procedure to the patient.
2. Place the patient in a comfortable position with the head supported.

3. Obtain a good light.
4. Sterilize the platinum loop by heating over a spirit lamp immediately before use. As platinum cools very quickly there is no danger of burning the patient.
5. He is instructed to look up and the sterilized loop is passed over the conjunctiva of the lower fornix in a continuous stroke from inner to outer canthus, the loop is then gently *stroked* onto a culture media (blood or chocolate agar), which has previously been labelled Right and Left eye. The loop is then re-sterilized and the same procedure is carried out for the other eye. It is necessary for the nurse to wear a mask during the procedure to prevent the culture plate from becoming contaminated.

The culture must be sent to the Bacteriological Department for incubation immediately it has been taken.

CUTTING EYELASHES

Equipment (Plate 11)

1 pair of Strabismus scissors
1 tube Vaseline
5–10 lint squares

This procedure is carried out as a routine prior to intraocular operations. In addition, it is sometimes carried out prior to operations on the lid margins and in cases of burns to the lids when the eyelashes themselves are burnt and crumbling into the eye. The patient should be reassured that the eyelashes *will regrow.*

Method

1. Explain the procedure to the patient.
2. Place the patient in a comfortable position with the head supported.
3. Obtain a good light.
4. *Lightly* grease the blades of the scissors. This will cause the eyelashes to adhere to them.
5. Ask the patient to close his eyes 'as though asleep' i.e. not to squeeze or screw-up the eyelids.
6. Slightly erect the upper lid and cut the lashes with a long continuous cut, not jerky snips. After each cut the blades should be wiped clean and re-greased. Always cut lashes about 1 mm from the lid margin to avoid any chance of snipping the lid should the patient move, not only would this be painful for the patient, but it would increase the risk of infection.
7. Ask the patient to look up above his head and pull down the excess skin of the lower lid into the infraorbital area, and turn the lashes of the lower lid in the same manner.
8. Wipe any excess grease off the lids and examine the eye to make sure that no lash has been left on the lids or conjunctiva. Some surgeons also ask for irrigation of the eye as a lash may inadvertently fall into the eye and not be

easily removed with a damp swab. Such a lash, if left on the eye, could cause a *corneal abrasion*.

LACRIMAL SYRINGING

Equipment (Plate 14)

1 Nettleship punctum dilator
1 lacrimal canula
1 2 ml syringe
1 gallipot
normal saline
5–10 lint squares
guttae Ophthaine 0.5% or amethocaine 1%

This procedure is generally performed to ascertain whether or not the lacrimal passages are patent.

Method

1. Explain the procedure to the patient.
2. Place the patient in a comfortable position with head supported either lying down or in a slightly recumbent position.
3. Instil guttae Ophthaine 0.5% or guttae amethocaine 1%.
4. A good light focused on the punctum is necessary.
5. Pour normal saline into the gallipot and fill the syringe, placing the canula onto the end, re-checking patency of the canula at the same time.
6. Expose the punctum of the lower lid by drawing the excess skin in a downward and slightly lateral direction to the infraorbital ridge with the second finger of the left or right hand. This will assist dilatation by stretching the canaliculus.
7. The thumb of the same hand may be used to hold a swab against the lower lid to prevent normal saline running down the patient's face if the lacrimal passage is blocked.
8. The Nettleship's dilator is held between the index finger and thumb. The point of the dilator is inserted into the punctum in a *slightly downward and then nasal direction*. A little pressure is applied and a slight twist of the dilator between thumb and index finger is made.
9. The dilator is withdrawn and the lacrimal canula with syringe attached is inserted in the same way as the dilator.
10. 3–4 mm. of saline is injected, but *not under pressure* as this could damage tissue.
11. The patient is asked if he can feel or taste anything in his throat and if so to swallow. In this case, the passages are considered to be *patent*. At the same time, the nurse observes whether the saline is being returned through the upper or lower punctum. When this occurs, the passage is considered blocked. In some cases, the nurse may observe saline being returned through either punctum and the patient will still state that he can feel or taste saline in his throat; the duct is considered to be *partially blocked*.

12. The result of the procedure is entered on the patient's notes and the surgeon informed.

TONOMETRY WITH SCHIÖTZ TONOMETER

Equipment (Plate 12)

1 Schiötz tonometer
guttae Ophthaine 0.5% or guttae butacaine 4%
lint squares
tonometric chart

TONOMETRY is carried out to record the intraocular tension i.e. the tension inside the eyeball. Although experience permits the surgeon or ophthalmic nurse to estimate intraocular tension by digital palpation, the only accurate method is tonometry. The most frequently and easily used apparatus is the Schiötz tonometer, although the most accurate is considered to be the Applanation tonometer. It has obvious disadvantages for General Ward use, but is very useful in the Outpatient Department.

Method

1. Assemble the tonometer and test its accuracy upon the metal testing disc.
2. Make the patient comfortable, lying down with his chin slightly elevated. This position must be maintained for it is necessary to have the cornea 'horizontal' for an accurate reading. The nurse stands behind the patient's head.
3. Instil two drops of local anaesthetic into each eye. The choice of the type of local anaesthetic is important as it must *not* be one which has an effect upon the pupil. Should two drops not be sufficient, one or two more can be added, but it is not practicable to double-pad the patient afterwards.
4. The patient is generally asked to hold up the index finger of the hand opposite th e eye to be tested and to focus upon it. The finger is adjusted by the nurse so that the patient is focusing with the eye correctly positioned.
5. The nurse gently draws the skin folds of the lids apart *over the orbital margins* with the 1st and 2nd fingers of the hand not holding the tonometer.
6. The tonometer is then placed very lightly and centrally upon the patient's cornea. Great care is taken *not* to move the tonometer while it is resting on the cornea as this will cause an abrasion.
7. The recording is registered mentally by the nurse, or jotted down upon a scrap pad, and the tonometer is removed. The recorded number is compared with the tonometer scale and then converted into mm Hg.
8. The same technique is adopted for the other eye.
9. When charting, the nurse should always use a red graph for the right eye and a black or blue one for the left eye.
10. A drop of Paroline is often instilled afterwards.
11. If the patient complains of pain a short while after the reading this may be due to abrasion of the cornea and must be treated according to its severity, with

either application of an antibiotic ointment alone or with the addition of a pad and bandage.

It is extremely important to cleanse the testing disc and the stylet end of the tonometer between each patient. An ether methylated spirit swab, flaming on a lamp, or phenylmercuric borate solution 1/32000 can be used; a modern trend is to use a very fine pre-sterilized plastic cap, 'Tonofilm', over the tonometer for each patient, which is then discarded after use. This is rather expensive and many people consider that the additional weight, light though it is, gives an inaccurate reading, however the 'Tonofilm' has its uses when dealing with an infected cornea.

Before the tonometer is put away, it must be dismantled and thoroughly cleansed. The weights are taken off and the plungers unscrewed and removed, a pipe cleaner dipped in methylated ether is then passed through the barrel. The weights and plunger are cleansed with a swab and the tonometer placed inside the velvet-lined case. It is a delicate precision instrument and must be handled with care.

CARBOLIZATION OF THE CORNEA

Equipment (Plate 16)

1 lid speculum
5 lint squares 5 cm × 5 cm
5 sharpened wooden applicators, sterile
5 triangular pieces of blotting paper, sterile
1 small drachm glass, gallipot or watch-glass
1 corneal loupe
1 Saunders needle, sterile. For surgeon's use only.
guttae cocaine 4%, fluorescein 1%, sodium chloride 0·9%,
Oc. atropine 1%, Ol. atropine 1%, Ol. hyoscine ¼%,
Oc. chloramphenicol 0·5%, carbolic acid, guttæ adrenaline 0·01%

Carbolization is sometimes performed as a treatment for a corneal ulcer.

Method

1. Explain the procedure to the patient.
2. Anaesthetize the patient's eye with 6–8 drops of guttae cocaine 4% in addition to guttae adrenaline 0·01%.
3. Place the patient in a comfortable lying position with the head supported.
4. Obtain a good light.
5. Insert a speculum to separate the eyelids.
6. Stain with guttae fluorescein to show exact area of corneal ulceration. Excess fluorescein is removed by sodium chloride 0·9% solution.
7. The surgeon may wish to curette the surface of the ulcer with a Saunders needle, before applying the carbolic.
8. The ulcer and surrounding cornea are dried with the blotting paper to prevent the carbolic from spreading over the rest of the cornea.
9. The sharpened tip of the wooden applicator is dipped in the carbolic. The

floor and edges of the ulcer are touched with carbolic and immediately turn white. Great care must be taken *not to touch the conjunctiva*, as severe pain would be experienced by the patient, and conjunctivitis would also result. Several applications of carbolic may be required, and *each time* the ulcer and surrounding area are dried with blotting paper. It is often useful to keep a swab or piece of blotting paper in the lower fornix to absorb any increased lacrimation which may occur.

10. Oc. atropine 1% is instilled before closing the eye. The ointment will have a soothing and lubricating effect while atropine will dilate the pupil and relax the ciliary muscle to prevent iritis. This carbolization is in effect an induced corneal abrasion and is treated as one.
11. A firm pad and bandage are applied.
12. Although carbolization is not a painful procedure, the patient may later experience some discomfort when the cocaine wears off and it is kinder to give, with the surgeon's permission, an analgesic such as Paracetamol or Codis afterwards.
13. It is desirable to re-examine the eye on the following day to ascertain its progress.

EVERTING THE EYE LIDS

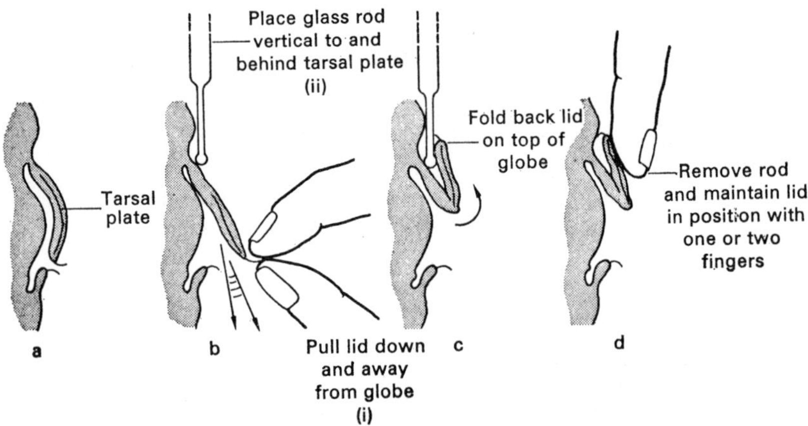

FIG 26 Eversion of the Upper Lid

As patients frequently present with conjunctival foreign bodies or conditions of the conjunctiva it is often necessary to expose the conjunctiva i.e.

A By eversion of the lower lid.

B By eversion of the upper lid.

C By eversion of lid to examine retrotarsal fold.

D By eversion of upper lid with one hand.

A nurse should *always practice upon an unaffected eye* in order to become proficient because when the need arises to carry out this procedure invariably the patient is suffering a great deal of discomfort and often pain.

(A) Lower lid

The patient is asked to look up, the lid is drawn down and with some manipulation all the folds of conjunctiva can be exposed.

(B) Upper lid

The anatomy of the lid must always be remembered notably that it contains the tarsal plate *which cannot be folded back upon itself* (fig. a) so great care and patience must be exercised when attempting to evert the lid.

The nurse may carry out this procedure whilst standing in front of, or behind the patient. It is advantageous to be conversant with both approaches particularly as there is a need to perform this procedure from behind or above whilst irrigating an eye.

1. Inform the patient that you are going to look underneath the eyelid and that although it could be uncomfortable it will not be painful.
2. Make the patient comfortable, either semi-recumbent in a chair or lying down with one pillow.
3. Focus an adequate light upon the eye.
4. Tip the patient's chin upwards to create an effective working angle.
5. Ask the patient to look down and to keep looking down to his feet.
6. With your forefinger and thumb grasp the eyelashes of the upper lid and gently pull it downwards and away from the globe—eyeball, this movement straightens out the excess skin fold above the tarsal plate (fig. b(i)).
7. Place a glass rod or finger perpendicular to and behind the tarsal plate (fig. b(ii)) and fold the lid back onto it (fig. c).
8. The rod can then be removed and the lid held by the index finger (fig. d).
9. When the examination has been completed ask the patient to look up, this will aid the lid to return to its normal position.

(C) Eversion of lid to examine retrotarsal fold. (Double Eversion)

Following the eversion of the upper lid some anaesthetic drops can be instilled and the retrotarsal fold can be exposed by placing a glass rod under the edge and lifting it as the rod is moved along. Encourage the patient to keep looking down.

(D) Eversion of upper lid with one hand

This procedure should only be undertaken by a very experienced nurse, even so the procedure is not a particularly comfortable one for the patient. Its use is limited to (a) patients who have had their eye lashes cut and (b) the possible need during irrigation of an eye.

16 *FIRST AID*

To avoid the risk of blindness, accidents to the eye require *the earliest possible attention*; the treatment can often be carried out immediately before removing the patient to an Ophthalmic Hospital or a General Practitioner. The treatments to be described are only FIRST AID, and if any difficulty or delay is experienced before being able to render such aid, the importance of medical care should come first.

Acid or Alkaline Burns

These, in common with various other liquids such as ammonia and hair lacquer, can all be treated in the same manner, although ideally acids and alkalines respond better to antidotes. Basically, the prime factor is to irrigate the eye *as quickly as possible, and to dilute or wash out the causative agent*; this can be done with warm tap water in an eye bath or egg cup, if only a small quantity was splashed into the eye; a teapot or small jug are ideal for home irrigation, if large quantities of water are required, while the patient holds his head sideways over a bowl. When the eye feels more comfortable, it should be covered with a clean handkerchief and the patient taken immediately to hospital.

If it is known that an acid or alkaline has been splashed into the eye, irrigation of the eye immediately with warm water is more important than searching for an antidote, this can always be used as a second irrigation. The commonest household antidote to an acid is sodium bicarbonate, 1 teaspoonful to ½ pint of water, and for an alkali, vinegar or boracic acid, again 1 teaspoonful to ½ pint of water. Corrosive burns can cause *symblepharon* (i.e. adhesion of the eyelid to the eyeball) if not promptly treated.

Black Eye

This is due to superficial bruising of the tissues in and around the lids following a blow. Frequently, no actual damage is accorded to the eye, but this very much depends upon the accompanying circumstances; for example, in road traffic accidents, impact from car windscreens can cause orbital fractures, broken glass can result in lacerated eyelids or even perforating wounds of the eyeball. These conditions will often be treated in hospital. Occasionally a blow from a champagne cork or a squash ball can cause a haemorrhage inside the eyeball or detachment of the retina; the patient usually complains of sudden loss of vision, partial or even extensive, and again medical aid must be sought immediately.

First Aid treatments that can be carried out are:

(a) Remove any obvious pieces of glass or grit that might be surrounding the eyes or be on the lids, and

(b) lightly apply cold compresses to the lids to reduce swelling of the tissues, and therefore enable the ophthalmologist to examine the eyes more easily.

Always seek medical aid if the lids become excessively oedematous, and the patient complains of pain or visual loss, even if the circumstances appear trivial.

Foreign Bodies

These fall into three main categories:

1. Conjunctival
2. Corneal
3. Subtarsal.

Should there be an obvious foreign body such as grit or an eyelash in the lower fornix, this can be removed with a corner of a clean handkerchief.

1. *Conjunctival and Lower Fornix*

The patient should be placed in a comfortable position with the head supported, an armchair is most useful, a good light is necessary. If there is any history or sign of dust being blown into the eye, irrigation of the eye is helpful, and further examination of the eye should then be made, in order that any remaining foreign bodies be removed before the patient is taken to hospital with his eye covered. This is a necessary procedure, as other foreign bodies can damage the cornea, *even without* the patient rubbing his eye; by the mere action of blinking or squeezing his eye, the patient can cause the foreign body to move.

2. *Corneal*

These should only be removed in hospital by a doctor or a trained experienced ophthalmic nurse. The Slit lamp is often used by the doctor while removing an embedded foreign body, although the use of a binocular loupe or magnifying spectacles is generally sufficient. It is therefore essential that, in the case of a corneal foreign body, the patient should be taken or advised to go to hospital. The eye should be covered and the patient instructed to keep his eye closed under the improvised pad to prevent further damage such as abrasion of the cornea by the pad.

3. *Subtarsal*

These are generally the easiest to remove and give immediate relief on removal. Having made the patient comfortable in an armchair, with the head supported and with a good light directed on the eye, evert the upper lid either with a matchstick or a finger. With a clean handkerchief, the corner of which has been dipped in water, the foreign body can be removed. Always make sure that there are *no smaller pieces left* on the other parts of the tarsal plate, and it is often wise to show the patient what you have removed.

Having dealt with a subtarsal foreign body and those of the conjunctiva and lower fornix, should the patient still complain of discomfort, again, take him to hospital for medical care as there may well be a *retained corneal foreign body* or a *corneal abrasion*, which would only be apparent if stained with fluorescein; in addition, cases of early conjunctivitis often begin with a 'gritty' feeling in the eye.

Lacerations of the Eyeball

These can occur to the conjunctiva, sclera and cornea, often as a result of road accidents, children playing with scissors or other pointed objects, etc. *All must be treated as if the eyeball itself has been perforated*, therefore cover the eye with lids closed to prevent infection and further damage and take the patient to hospital immediately; avoid pressure on the injured eye.

Laceration of the Eyelids

Any superficially retained cause of the laceration e.g. glass particle should be removed and the eye covered, with the lids closed in the most natural position possible, and the patient immediately taken to hospital. As with any laceration around the eye, the risk of perforating injury must never be overlooked. The complications that can result from an often apparently simple laceration are very serious. A wound of the lower lid may (a) involve the canaliculus and subsequent scar tissue can block the lacrimal passages, (b) lead to abnormalities of the lid margin and regrowth of eyelashes towards the cornea. Laceration of the upper lid may also damage the levator palpebrae superioris muscle and result in ptosis (drooping of the upper lid).

Lime Burns

These may occur to workmen on building sites or children playing on and around the site. Cement powder contains a proportion of lime. A lime burn can cause most serious scarring of the cornea, *with permanent damage* to the sight so it is essential to administer adequate and immediate treatment. *Little effective treatment can be performed at home*. The obvious pieces should be wiped away. If possible, the eyes should be irrigated and liquid paraffin or even olive oil applied to the cornea. Often, this is impossible; because of severe pain the patient cannot co-operate. The eyes should be covered, and the patient taken to hospital *without delay*.

Caustic Soda Burns

These are commonly caused by household cleaning agents as caustic soda is a constituent of many. As with all other burns previously mentioned, these should be dealt with promptly and effectively in the above manner.

Subconjunctival Haemorrhage

Subconjunctival haemorrhage may not always be as innocent as it appears and should always be treated with caution. Medical advice should be sought. If associated with trauma, always cover the eye and take the patient to hospital.

17 *SURGICAL NURSING CARE*

Pre- and Post-Operative Nursing Care

An intraocular operation is one in which an incision is made into the eye.

There are many points common to the nursing care of all patients undergoing intraocular operations. *They will be dealt with in detail in the pre- and post-operative nursing care of lens extraction,* and will not necessarily be repeated in the ensuing descriptions of the nursing care of glaucoma, keratoplasty, and retinal detachment. Only the main principles of each will be outlined.

CATARACT EXTRACTION

There is no known treatment other than surgical intervention for the removal of a cataract.

Pre-operative Care

Admission is preferable 48 hours prior to operation. This is because of the need for: (1) Orientation, (2) Investigation of general health, (3) Preparation of the eye.

(1) *Orientation*

The patient is often elderly and practically blind and therefore takes longer to become accustomed to the ward and nursing staff.

On admission it is important to tell the patient and his relatives what treatment he will be receiving for the immediate post-operative period. Both must be familiar with visiting hours. As the patient will have a soft diet at first, relatives must be asked not to bring in food which is hard to bite e.g. biscuits and apples. At this stage, it should be noted if the patient has any special dietary requirements for medical or religious reasons. Enquiries about financial problems, if any, tactfully made, will often prevent post-operative worry, as will enquiries regarding home conditions, so that convalescence may be arranged if necessary. It must be realised that many elderly patients live alone in often difficult housing situations i.e. long flights of stairs, inconvenient toilet facilities. If, for one reason or another, relatives or friends are unable to give assistance during the two weeks' home convalescence period, the social worker will require to make convalescent home arrangements or, failing that, the use of the Meals on Wheels, Home Help or Social Visiting services. If the patient has other problems, family, housing, work, or any special pending commitments he should be referred to the social worker for help. In many cases, the social worker will have seen the patient as an out-patient prior to admission to hospital.

At this time, it is advisable to discourage smoking both before operation and for the next few days after. The patient must be told to what extent he will be confined to bed and when he will receive aperients. This particular aspect invariably causes great worry to the elderly patient. If unaccustomed to a bedpan or urinal he should be taught how to use them, how to co-operate with lifting in bed, how to summon nursing aid by the use of the bell, and how to drink through a straw or, if necessary, to use a feeding cup. The importance of deep breathing and leg exercises should be stressed.

All these things must be discussed in order to gain the patient's full confidence and co-operation.

(2) *Investigation of General Health*

By virtue of age alone, these patients are fortunate indeed if they are in completely good health. Whereas signs of any specific illness may not be apparent, simple urine testing may show latent diabetes, or the recording of an abnormal blood pressure may have to be investigated. Obvious signs, such as a nervous disability, may preclude the use of a local anaesthetic, or chronic bronchitis may suggest a course of prophylactic treatment or even postponement of the operation until summer.

Should no abnormality present itself, the recording of the weight, T.P.R., blood pressure and urinalysis on admission always serves as a useful guide for comparison during the immediate post-operative period. Any drugs that the patient may have been prescribed by his general practitioner are generally maintained and noted. Any known drug allergies are noted both on his medication sheet and on his medical notes.

Routine investigations such as haemoglobin and chest X-ray are ordered at the discretion of the surgeon.

(3) *Preparation of the Eye*

The eyelashes of the appropriate eye are cut (see page 108).

Syringing of the lacrimal passages is carried out only at the request of some surgeons to make sure that the tear duct is patent, or if the eye appears sticky and if any obvious epiphora is noted.

A conjuctival culture is taken from both eyes (see page 107).

The instillation of prophylactic drops can now be commenced. Guttae chloramphenicol 0.5% is currently the drug of choice being a broad spectrum antibiotic. These drops are instilled three times a day to both eyes.

On the day before operation, a mild aperient such as 'Milpar' (liquid paraffin and magnesium hydroxide) 15–30 ml is given if required.

A mild sedative, such as dichloralphenazone 650–1300 mg, is given the night before the operation. Barbiturates are generally not suitable for the elderly patient.

On the morning of the operation, the patient is given a bath. The hair of female patients is combed and plaited, if long. Male patients are encouraged to shave as they are generally not allowed to do so for several days post-operatively.

The culture report is checked, and if pathogenic organisms are present the operation may have to be postponed.

Shortly before the premedication is due, the patient is encouraged to go to the toilet and then to change into an operation gown. If the operation is to be performed under a general anaesthetic, dentures are removed and placed in a labelled carton. If the operation is to be performed under a local anaesthetic, dentures may be left in if the patient so wishes, *provided they are well fitting*; should this be doubtful, they should be removed because a patient can become very drowsy while under premedication and the dentures easily slip into the back of the throat and cause obstruction. If dentures are left in, they should not be removed until after the first dressing.

The patient is put to bed on a divided theatre canvas, as this is easier to remove. If these are not available, a plain operating canvas may be used covered with a draw sheet. The draw sheet is required for the patient's comfort, for, in this instance, the canvas will have to be left in position until after the first dressing.

The patient is premedicated, according to the type of anaesthetic. At this stage, a label which has been signed by the house surgeon stating patient's name, age and eye for operation is fixed to the patient's wrist. Some surgeons like the pupil to be fully dilated before lens extraction, this necessitates the intensive instillation of mydriatics for about forty-five minutes prior to operation. Other surgeons prefer the pupil to be only partially dilated, in this case either homatropine 1% b.d. is instilled from the time of admission or homatropine 2% with cocaine 2% is instilled immediately before operation.

If the operation is to be performed under a local anaesthetic, guttae cocaine 4%, adrenaline 0·1%, homatropine 1% and chloramphenicol 0·5% are instilled every minute for five minutes and then at five minute intervals until operation. Note guttae atropine is not prescribed because its action is irreversible. A patient should not receive more than two drops of adrenaline 0·1% and more than 6–8 drops of cocaine 4%. If desired, more can be instilled in theatre. During this period, the eye must be covered, either by a pad or lint flap, to protect the anaesthetised cornea. If an eye pad is used, great care must be taken to ensure that *the eye is closed under it to prevent an abrasion of the cornea.*

The frequency, type and percentage of all drops are naturally ordered by the surgeon, and the above is only to serve as *a general indication of what may be used.*

It is wise when instilling the drops to have prepared a list of times when all drops are due so that they may be ticked off after each instillation. The two nurses checking the premedication must check all drops with the treatment sheet, leaving the drops in their rack at the patient's bedside for successive instillations.

The patient is accompanied to the theatre by a nurse, the label on his wrist having been checked by Sister or Staff Nurse before he leaves the ward. The nurse will remain in the anaesthetic room until he is either anaesthetised or the local anaesthetic has been given. Whenever possible, the nurse should accompany the patient into the theatre in order that she may see as much of the operation as possible and to have a better understanding of the type of nursing care required of her. Should the patient have a local anaesthetic, it is very comforting for him to hold the nurse's hand.

Even with modern anaesthesia, the surgeon frequently prefers to perform the operation under local anaesthetic. From a post-operative nursing point of view, this is also advantageous as the patient is able to co-operate, less likely to become restless and can often sit up on returning to the ward. When a general anaesthetic is given, most surgeons give a facial nerve block of local anaesthetic to prevent the patient from squeezing his eye while recovering from the anaesthetic.

Post-operative Care

The patient is returned to the ward with one eye covered by an eye pad, cartella shield and bandage. The divided canvas is removed. Unless a general anaesthetic has been given or an air bubble injected into the anterior chamber, he should be made comfortable with two or three pillows *supporting the head, neck and shoulders,* When the patient is more awake, he may sit up higher with the back rest extended. a locker placed *on the side of the uncovered eye,* his head well supported, a drink poured out and placed within reach, while he should be given *a bell* with which to summon a nurse.

When a general anaesthetic has been administered all care regarding a patient regaining consciousness must be taken and particular attention paid to prevent the patient knocking his eye. If the patient becomes very restless the anaesthetist should be informed. If the patient becomes nauseated the prescribed drug e.g. perphanazine 4–5 mg, must be immediately given to obviate vomiting as this could result in damage to the eye. This drug is generally to be avoided in young adults. Dichloralphenazone may be used each night as a sedative.

Pain is unusual although a mild analgesic, such as 'Codis', may be given if required at any time.

As with any surgical wound, the aim of post-operative nursing care is to promote healing. An intraocular incision usually takes 5–6 days to heal. This may be delayed depending on the patient's age and general health.

Details of specific nursing care will, of course, be upheld conscientiously but, in addition, the nurse must be constantly alert to any circumstances which are adverse to her patient's recovery.

A quiet and happy ward is of great importance. Unnecessary noise of crockery, door banging and movement of chairs, etc., may startle a patient who may then unconsciously squeeze his eye. Also, an unhappy patient will become anxious and restless.

Patients in older age groups may cling to their independence and others may not wish to cause extra work for the nursing staff and, in so doing, attempt feats which may result in injury to the eye.

The nurse must therefore give constant care and attention to all the needs of her patient in such a manner that he does not feel suffocated by care or that he is causing unnecessary work.

Position

The patient should sit up or lie flat with one pillow but in no circumstances on the side. His locker remains on the side of the unoperated eye so that movement of the head will be towards that side.

Approach

The nurse must always approach the patient from the unoperated side to minimise the movement of the patient's head. In addition the nurse must always let the patient be aware of her approach by addressing him in a quiet manner before touching him, moving his bed or locker, etc. When talking to a patient who is either blind or double-padded, the nurse should make a point of holding the patient's hand so that he knows in which direction to address his reply. There is nothing worse for the patient than to be addressed *by an impersonal voice from some unknown position.*

Washing

Until the first dressing has been performed, only the patient's hands and round the mouth are washed, the pre-operative bath having dispensed with the necessity for a thorough and early post-operative wash. Mouth rinses are also given but teeth must not be brushed.

After the first dressing there is usually nothing to prevent the patient rinsing his own hands and face under observation. This gives a certain feeling of independence. A daily blanket bath is also given by the nursing staff.

Pressure Areas

These are treated by rolling the patient towards the unoperated eye. It has been argued that this involves too much movement and that two nurses should lift the patient whilst the third treats his pressure areas. With this method, the condition of the pressure areas cannot be observed and three nurses are not always available.

Lifting

The usual method of lifting a patient i.e. with his head forward, is not particularly good for his eye. It is best for nurses to help the patient to sit forward and support himself with his hands behind him on the bed. The pillows may then be arranged and the bedclothes turned back. The patient is asked to bend his knees and is then lifted back. Patients in the prone position can often best be helped by bending their knees, placing one arm around the waist of a nurse on each side of the bed and lifted along in this manner.

Hair

As previously stated, the hair of a female patient, if long, is best plaited as it may then be left uncombed for several days. A comb may be passed through the hair close to the head after the first dressing but pulling at tangles and complicated dressing of the hair should be avoided.

Shaving

The male patient is not allowed to be shaved until the third post-operative day and it is wiser to employ the hospital barber to shave him until the sixth day or even later still should the patient not manage himself.

Diet

This has already been discussed with the patient in the pre-operative period. It should be light and not require much biting or chewing. The choice should be varied as soft foods can often be monotonous. Notice must be taken of all food brought in by visitors as this can often be contrary to the dietary needs of the patient. A normal diet is usually given after the third day.

Feeding

The patient must be fed until the first dressing has been performed. However, if this is satisfactory he may then feed himself. The use of a bed table just below eye level, food that has been cut up and an attentive nurse are all useful aids in helping the patient to maintain some independence. If feeding himself causes undue movement it should be discouraged and he should be fed.

Feeding patients with afternoon tea is a comparatively easy matter as the patient is able to hold sandwiches and cake himself. Meals entailing the use of cutlery of course need extra care. The nurse must remember that life for a patient being fed can be extremely monotonous especially if he is unable to see with his other eye. Her encouragement and imagination can go a long way towards making what could be a boring necessity for the patient into a pleasant occasion.

The nurse should stand at the side of the bed opposite the operated eye. Soup from a cup or feeder can often be managed by the patient. He should be offered a drink of water before commencing each course, his meal should be described to him and he should be asked if he would like a little of everything on the spoon or fork at the same time. He should also be asked if he has any preference for being fed with a spoon or a fork. The nurse should be fully proficient with either.

The ophthalmic patient is not generally ill in the accepted sense. In fact, he is often more alert than the great majority of patients and sometimes resents the necessity for being fed, but asking the patient to make a choice in these matters does help to restore some feeling of independence.

The nurse must give the patient time to swallow each mouthful before offering another, and warn him when he is nearing the end of each course. An imaginative nurse will usually talk to the patient during mealtimes, *keeping to topics which do not require his verbal participation.*

For patients in the upright position, a cup or glass is generally managed satisfactorily but the addition of a 'Flexostraw' is helpful. Patients lying down can use a feeding cup and tilt it themselves to avoid the risk of coughing if the drink is given too quickly. Some patients experience difficulty in using a feeding cup, and a straw passed through the spout makes it easier to use. Two points to observe when giving a patient a drink from a feeding cup are (1) that the spout is not chipped and (2) that the cup is only half-filled. An over-filled cup will spill liquid over the patient when he tilts it to drink.

Aperients

It will already have been explained to the patient on admission that because of his soft diet and inactivity it will be unlikely that he will have his bowels open for 3–4 days and that this temporary constipation *will cause him no harm.* Milpar 30–60 ml daily and three times a day on the third day post-operatively generally achieves satisfactory results. Glycerin suppositories can be used should the 'Milpar' prove ineffective. The use of a sani-chair on the third day is also an advantage. These measures are taken to (a) prevent worry by the patient which could cause restlessness, (b) prevent straining to pass a constipated stool, (c) prevent the difficulty and distress that the patient experiences when using a bedpan.

Smoking

This is often a problem. A patient who cannot see presents a real fire risk when smoking in bed. Where possible, smoking is entirely discouraged but, if this is obviously going to be impracticable, it is much better to allow smoking at certain times, such as after meals and when tea is served, so that the nurse can light the cigarette or pipe for the patient.

A small point to note pre-operatively is that if a patient makes his own cigarettes he should be encouraged to prepare a supply to last him throughout his post-operative period.

Visitors should be asked, in the patient's interest, to refrain from smoking. In fact, in most hospitals they are forbidden to do so, particularly as visiting hours are now more extensive and frequent than in the past.

Visiting Hours

Visiting hours are frequently under discussion. The patient's need for mental diversion and the pleasure obtained from seeing relatives and friends must not be overlooked. On the other hand, the need of the post-operative ophthalmic patient for rest and quiet must not be forgotten. In addition, the majority are elderly and prolonged visiting hours can cause great strain and be very tiring. It is considered best to restrict visitors until after the first dressing and, following this, to allow daily visiting for short periods in the afternoon and evening. This has the advantage of not tiring the patient and enabling him to have a greater variety of visitors. It is often wise not to allow babies or very young children to visit because of the risk of noise leading to sudden movement by the patient. In addition grandparents frequently wish to bend over to kiss the child and this again is a risk as even a small baby can cause damage to the eye by the sudden movement of a hand.

Night Care

The nurse must be particularly attentive during the night as less staff are on duty and sometimes elderly patients become a little confused. This is now a less frequent occurrence than in the past, partly due to the restrained use of barbiturates and partly because most surgeons now cover only one eye after operation. Great care should be taken to settle the patient comfortably for the night, a bedpan given, draw sheet straightened, pillows arranged, back rest removed and a warm milk drink given with the night sedation. This is usually dichloralphenazone 650 mg to 1300 mg. Male patients should have a urinal within reach, and the nurse should make sure that patients have a bedside bell and a drink within easy reach. This attention and a maintained quiet throughout the night by the nurse should ensure that the patient spends an undisturbed night.

On rare occasions the elderly patient can become restless and it may be necessary to use padded cot-sides to contain him in bed, particularly if he becomes forgetful of his surroundings or is temporarily confused.

Ambulation

Although surgeons vary as to when they consider it advisable for patients to be allowed up, provided there are no obvious contra-indications and great care is exercised by the nursing staff, the patient is usually allowed up for bedmaking after the first dressing.

The nurse must make quite sure that the patient does not bend over in an attempt to put on his slippers, etc., and that he is gently helped from his bed. He must be told to feel behind him for the arms of the chair and then to gently lower himself into it.

It is important that the patient does not bend over to feel for the chair or sit down suddenly in it as both of these movements could lead to an iris prolapse. At this stage the patient is *reminded* that he must summon a nurse should he wish anything retrieved from the floor. If the patient is very restless in bed, sitting in a chair for long periods throughout the day is preferable to constant wriggling around the bed. Pressure areas can be treated with less movement of the patient and post-operative complications such as chest conditions and deep venous thrombosis are more easily avoided.

The patient is generally allowed to use the sani-chair by his bedside on the third day. On the sixth day he is encouraged to take short gentle walks with help, and also to have meals sitting at his bedside. From the seventh day onwards he is allowed up with care for most of the day and also a general bath is allowed provided the eye is covered by a pad and bandage.

It cannot be overstressed that the nurse must be constantly aware of her patient's needs and be ready to render any necessary assistance.

First Dressing

Equipment

Top of Trolley: 1 sterile pack containing 10–15 5 cm × 5 cm lint squares or dressed orange sticks
2 eye pads
2 cartella shields, one right and one left

1 dressing towel or paper tissue
1 hand towel
1 gallipot
1 pair straight iris scissors
1 pair Moorfields suture forceps
1 sterile jug containing normal saline, placed in
1 bowl, containing warm water to take chill off normal saline

Bottom of Trolley: Prescribed drops and ointments
patient's eye medication sheet
1 examination torch
Sellotape in dispenser
5 mm 'Kling' bandage
dressing scissors in container
disposable bag to receive soiled dressings
1 container to receive soiled instruments

Method

1. Explain the procedure to the patient.
2. Draw blinds over the windows to reduce direct light upon the patient.
3. Standing on the side of the operated eye, remove one or two pillows from behind the patient. The semi-recumbent position allows drops to remain in the eye more easily.
4. Prepare lengths of Sellotape or strapping, approximately 15 centimetres long to hold an eye pad and cartella shield, and two pieces 2·5 centimetres long to fasten the bandage. These may all be attached by 6 mm to the patient's bedtable, and within reach of the dresser. Remove the outside wrapper from bandage, check drops and ointment with medication sheet, unscrewing the bottle caps and aspirating a drop into the pipette.
5. Place the patient's hands beneath the bedclothes as an added reminder for him not to touch his eye during the dressing.
6. Remove the bandage. With a 'Kling' disposable bandage this can be done by cutting it in front of the ear, and again where it crosses the patient's forehead. The patient then only needs to lift his head for a moment whilst the bandage is lifted off.
7. The strapping holding the eye pad is cut and this is also removed, providing that it is not adherent to the lids in which case it is left until the sterile dressing packet has been undone. As most surgeons place a piece of 'Tullegras' under the eye pad in theatre, this seldom occurs.
8. The outer wrapper of the sterile dressing packet is undone.
9. The dresser thoroughly washes her hands, rinses them in a skin cleansing solution such as benzalkonium 0·2% with chlorhexidine 0·04% or chlorhexidine 0·5% in 70% spirit and dries them on a sterile towel. This method of preparation has been devised in order to do without a second nurse.

Obviously, where an assistant is available these preparations can be done by her while the dresser is washing her hands.

10. The inner dressing packet is opened and the lint squares are separated and folded into four with the fluffy side inwards.
11. Normal saline is poured into the gallipot. A towel is draped around the side of the patient's head.
12. If the pad is stuck it is peeled off from above downwards, the lid being held by a moistened swab.
13. The lid sutures are cut close to the lid and the suture withdrawn using forceps. It is then cut close to the cheek where it has been attached with Sellotape. (These lid sutures are necessary due to the paralysis of the lids caused by the injection of lignocaine around the 7th nerve.)
14. The unoperated eye is bathed. The patient must be warned of this or he is likely to think a mistake has been made. The reason for this procedure is twofold: firstly, it gives the patient an idea of what to expect when his operated eye is bathed, thus ensuring his co-operation and, secondly, as there is always a certain amount of lacrimation of the other eye, the patient may find it difficult to open.
15. The operated eye is bathed, care being taken to remove excess grease from the 'Tullegras' and ointment.
16. The patient is asked to open both eyes and a swab is held on the lower lid of the operated eye to catch the overflow of tears which often occurs when the eye is opened for the first time.
17. When the patient has become accustomed to having both eyes open, the dresser may then shine the light from her inspection torch slowly across the unoperated eye onto the operated eye, at the same time holding the lids apart with the index finger on the upper lid and a swab under the thumb on the lower lid.

The eye must always be examined in the following methodical manner at every dressing until the patient has been discharged:

(a) The lids must be inspected to note any swelling or tenderness. This could be indicative of an allergy to the previously used drops or ointments or of an infection.

(b) If the lashes are encrusted or turn inwards, they must be carefully cleansed and stroked outwards.

(c) The conjunctiva may be excessively injected (red) or chemotic. This may also be a sign of drug allergy or of infection.

(d) The cornea should be bright and clear. Keratitis, iritis or infection may cause a cornea to be cloudy.

(e) The anterior chamber should have reformed and be clear. If the iris is pressed close to the cornea a shallow anterior chamber is present. A shallow anterior chamber can lead to the formation of anterior synechiae (see glossary, page 144). Mydriatic drops are normally instilled at the first dressing and dilatation of the pupil is maintained at subsequent dressings. The addition of a firm pad and bandage to press the edges of the section together and to prevent leakage from the section is also advantageous in reforming an anterior chamber.

A choroidal detachment can occur in the immediate post-operative period or even after the patient is discharged. Although it is not the nurse's responsibility to diagnose this condition it is usually manifest by a shallow or flat anterior chamber, often accompanied by the patient complaining of clouding of vision or even partial visual loss, both of which are reported to the surgeon. The choroid usually becomes re-attached in a comparatively short time with the aid of a firm pad and bandage. The surgeon may decide to drain off the fluid and restore the anterior chamber with an air bubble if the detachment persists and the anterior chamber remains flat.

Should the anterior chamber not be clear, it should be noted whether a hyphaema or a hypopyon is present. Hyphaema is usually due to bleeding from the iris or the edges of the corneo-scleral incision. It can be caused by a knock on the eye, cheek or forehead. It may also be spontaneous, diabetic patients are more prone to hyphaema. The patient usually experiences some pain and will often notice some clouding of vision. It can be quickly absorbed but may cause secondary glaucoma or staining of the cornea if absorption is delayed.

If a hyphaema is present, its appearance i.e. clotted or fluid and amount should be noted. It may not always be sufficient to fill the anterior chamber and gradually subsides forming a fluid level. It is then described accordingly e.g. total, two-thirds, half or crescentic. If the hyphaema is small and clotted with no signs of fresh haemorrhage, the patient may remain ambulant, but should there be any signs of further bleeding, a firm pad and bandage is applied and the patient must remain in bed with the head kept still. Analgesics may be given if required and heat can be applied with a Maddox heater but *not* by hot spoon bathings.

If a hypopyon is present it is usually sterile. Nevertheless, it is always treated in the early stages as if infected. A conjunctival culture is taken and intensive local drops, such as chloramphenicol 0·5%, are instilled every minute for 5 minutes, then every 5 minutes for one hour and then hourly, accompanied by systemic antibiotics and a mydriatic. Should the culture report be sterile and no change in the hypopyon be noted, steroids *may* then be indicated.

(f) The pupil should be central and its size noted. If there is an irregularity of the pupil above, thus giving it a pear-shaped appearance, the section is examined closely as this distortion is often indicative of iris prolapse.

(g) The section should be flat, without any suspicion of leaking aqueous or iris prolapse i.e. iris herniated into the corneo-scleral wound. If this has occurred, it is usually treated surgically by abscission of the prolapsed iris.

Excessive lacrimation should be noted although post-operatively this is not unusual; however, a small foreign body or drug allergy will also cause severe lacrimation.

If any of the above abnormalities appear, their presence should be immediately drawn to the attention of the surgeon.

If all is satisfactory, the prescribed drops can be instilled, great care being taken to see that the patient does not squeeze his eye. The dresser will use the hand with which she held her torch to hold the eye dropper, and again this hand is used for picking up the Sellotape, keeping the other hand clean to hold a swab to hold the lids apart and to take the eye pad and cartella shield from the trolley.

The patient is asked to gently close his eyes, and a fresh pad is applied followed by the cartella shield. The ends of the Sellotape fixing the pad and shield should terminate on top of each other so that the patient is not subjected to pieces of Sellotape all over his forehead and cheek. At each dressing the end pieces are left attached so that the patient's skin does not become sore by daily removal and unnecessary squeezing of the eye.

The patient's hair is tidied and the bandage re-applied, pillows are replaced and the patient is made comfortable. The nurse then washes her hands.

Where several eye dressings are to be performed from one trolley, the complete pre-sterilized dressing pack is of great advantage. They can be placed in a container on top of the trolley with a further container on the bottom of the trolley to receive instruments and gallipots. As with all surgical dressings, the more recently operated eyes are dressed first with intraocular cases taking precedence and any infected dressings, such as dacryocystitis, blepharitis, etc., kept until last.

Without alarming the patient and his relatives, the nurse should instruct the patient to take things quietly for at least two weeks after discharge. Stress should be laid upon the avoidance of bending, lifting heavy objects, travelling on buses or tube trains as far as possible. This emphasises the importance of ascertaining on admission the patient's home conditions and whether it may be considered necessary to send him to a convalescent home for this two week period. If the patient is staying with relatives, clear instructions should be given regarding the extent of his activities and although instructions are written upon all drops to be used, it is wise to repeat them with the patient and his relatives. If the patient is going home to be helped by the 'Meals on Wheels' and 'Home Help' Service, it is important to *teach him how to instil his own drops before leaving hospital.*

General complications which can occur

1. Chest complications
2. Deep venous thrombosis
3. Retention of urine
4. Post-operative mental confusion.

1. Chest complications are more rare than in the past due to the early ambulation of the patient. As previously stated, operations on chronic bronchitics are generally left until the spring or summer months and all patients are taught

deep breathing exercises pre-operatively; these are encouraged by the nursing staff post-operatively. Nevertheless, the nurse must be aware of the possibility of bronchitis, hypostatic pneumonia and pulmonary emboli.

2. Deep venous thrombosis also rarely occurs because of early ambulation and the teaching of leg exercises pre-operatively. Any complaint of pain in the calves by the patient must immediately be reported to the surgeon, a crepe supporting bandage applied to the legs and the patient put back to bed with the foot of the bed elevated. Medication may be ordered by the surgeon.
3. Retention of urine. This occurs more frequently in the male and is usually associated with an enlarged prostate gland. Information on nocturnal frequency or other such difficulties is generally obtained when enquiring about the patient's general health and will be treated before ophthalmic surgery is undertaken.

   If the condition is due to post-operative nervousness or associated with general anaesthesia, it is often helpful if the surgeon will allow him to stand out of bed to use his urinal. Occasionally, a relaxant drug, such as chlorpromazine hydrochloride, is prescribed to help the patient over the initial phase. Catheterisation is resorted to if other measures fail.
4. Post-operative mental confusion. This condition is also less common than it used to be. Forgetfulness in strange surroundings and routine i.e. waking up and not knowing where one is, is not to be confused with a true rambling disorientation. Understanding, reassurance, comfort, peace and a quiet manner by the nurse can frequently prevent further confusion by the patient. The first signs of restlessness, particularly nocturnal, confused speech or volubility should be reported. Should reassurance fail, these patients are sometimes sedated, or if slightly co-operative allowed to sit in an armchair for long periods. If these measures are not effective, they are frequently sent home before the full post-operative period is completed and their more familiar surroundings produce the desired effect of normality. A large proportion of these patients have surprisingly good visual results in spite of their excursions, and often inexperienced junior nurses may well question the necessity for the normal painstaking routine care.

The patient's post-operative care is ordered by the surgeon and, of course, this varies with the individual needs of each patient, but in the training of nurses it is necessary to have an accepted basic routine and, therefore, a brief guide of daily post-operative care to meet these needs is suggested.

1st post-operative day

1. Morning wash of hands and around mouth only. Mouth rinsed carefully but teeth not cleaned, dentures remain in. Back powdered, only with patient lifted not rolled, pressure areas as such are not treated until after first dressing.
2. Bed tidied and draw sheet pulled through if divided canvas has been used.
3. Fed with breakfast.
4. Milpar 30–60 ml O.D. is given if required.

5. *First dressing performed.*
6. Blanket bath given.
7. Patient may feed himself. Patient is allowed up for bed-making.
8. Afternoon and evening pressure areas are treated by rolling patient towards un-operated eye.
9. Deep breathing and leg exercises every four hours.
10. Eye treatment: guttae atropine 1%, oculentum chloramphenicol 0·5% and oculentum atropine 1% daily with added mydriasis as required by the surgeon.

2nd post-operative day

1. Blanket bath and up for bed-making in morning.
2. Teeth may be brushed carefully.
3. Dentures can be taken out to be cleaned. Remaining days as for 1st.

3rd post-operative day

1. May use Sani-chair by bedside.
2. Men may be shaved.
3. Milpar t.d.s. if required.

4th post-operative day

As 3rd.

1. 'Sennakot' 2 tablets at night if required.
2. Allowed to toilet in Sani-chair.
3. Length of time sitting in armchair increasing daily.

5th post-operative day

Women may wear their own nightdress.

6th post-operative day

1. Dark glasses may be worn.
2. Cartella shield at night.
3. Normal diet.
4. Up by bedside for meals
5. Short walks with help.
6. Guttae increased to:
   guttae atropine 1% b.d.
   guttae chloramphenicol 0·5% } t.d.s.
   guttae hydrocortisone 0·5% } t.d.s.

7th and 8th post-operative day

1. General bath taken with help. Pad and bandage applied to eye first.
2. Increased activity but no bending or stooping.
3. Transport arranged for discharge.

9th post-operative day

1. Removal of conjunctival suture if necessary.
2. Patient may wear own glasses with lens of operated eye occluded.

10th post-operative day

Discharge. Advice:

1. No stooping or lifting.
2. No hair washing for 2 weeks.
3. No public transport.
4. Always put in the prescribed drops for operated eye.
5. Inform own doctor if eye becomes painful or misty.

Give:

1. Out-patient follow up appointment, 2 weeks approximately.
2. Drops for use after discharge.

GLAUCOMA

Most patients admitted for drainage operations suffer from diminished vision to a greater or lesser extent. They have already been told that an operation is necessary to prevent further loss of vision *or* to maintain the status quo. The patients are often worried in case, as a result of the operation, they may lose what vision they have. For this reason, they need to be constantly reassured that this is not so, but at the same time it must be gently impressed upon them that the vision already lost *will not be regained.* This to some patients, is a great disappointment as most expect a dramatic result from an operation.

Pre-operative Nursing Care

Admission is forty-eight hours prior to operation, and preparation is as for lens extraction. All miotic drops in the eye to be operated on are continued until the immediate pre-operative period and, of course, will be continued post-operatively in the *unoperated* eye if previously prescribed. Any diuretics such as acetazolamide or dichlorphenamide will also be maintained pre-operatively unless the surgeon instructs otherwise, but they are generally discontinued post-operatively. Tonometry readings are taken at the request of the surgeon, often four hourly, but maybe less, depending on the intraocular pressure.

Pre-operative drops consist of:

guttae pilocarpine 1%–2%
guttae cocaine 4%
guttae chloramphenicol 0·5%
} Every five minutes for forty minutes.

Although it is an advantage for the surgeon to have a white eye to operate on, guttae adrenaline 0·1% is usually only instilled at ten minute intervals or sometimes even less frequently, lest it cause dilatation of the pupil.

Various drainage operations can be performed. The principle is basically the same, namely that of creating an artificial drainage channel at the corneo-scleral margin communicating with the filtration angle and through which the aqueous may drain subconjunctivally, thus relieving the intraocular tension.

Post-operative Nursing Care

The routine is less rigid than for lens extraction or keratoplasty because the incision is smaller and therefore there is less risk of complications.

At the first dressing, the depth of the anterior chamber must be noted; it may remain quite shallow for several days.

Guttae atropine 1% is usually prescribed post-operatively for the operated eye to prevent iritis and of course this will help to prevent possible posterior synechiae.

Additional mydriasis is generally prescribed for the operation of Anterior Flap Sclerotomy as this is a combined drainage operation and quite a large drainage bleb is commonly formed under the conjunctiva. The iris is additionally included in the corneo-scleral section and consequently the prevention of iritis is very important. A prophylactic measure against iritis usually taken by the surgeon at the end of the operation is a subconjunctival injection of methylprednisolone acetate ('Depomedrone').

Should the patient be receiving miotics to his other eye it is extremely important that, when the mydriatic is to be instilled into the operated eye, *it is checked by two nurses*. The danger of inducing an acute attack of glaucoma in the unoperated eye by the incorrect instillation of a mydriatic must not be underestimated or overlooked.

Some surgeons prescribe massage to the eye when the eye is dressed to encourage the drainage of aqueous humour. This entails the patient looking down and gentle but firm massage with the first and second *fingertips*. The patient is taught to do this himself before discharge. The massage is usually prescribed two to three times daily.

Complications are rare and seldom serious. The two most commonly seen are:

1. There may be a persistent aqueous leak resulting in a shallow anterior chamber.
   A firm pad and bandage is usually applied as a first measure, but if it persists a conjunctival fold is brought down over the drainage bleb.
2. Choroidal detachment, as described in lens extraction.

The patient is allowed to become ambulant as soon as the anterior chamber is reasonably well formed. The first five days are as for lens extraction.

6th day

1. Dark glasses may be worn.
2. Guttae increased from guttae atropine 1% and guttae chloramphenicol 0·5% to:
   guttae atropine 1% b.d.
   guttae chloramphenicol 0·5% } t.d.s.
   guttae prednisolone 0.5% }
   Again these drops are a guide only and may be increased or decreased by the surgeon.
3. Meals may be taken by bedside.
4. Conjunctival suture removed.
5. Cartella shield worn at night.

7th day

1. Up with care.
2. General bath with pad and bandage applied.
3. Patient taught to massage his eye.

8th day

Discharge.

Give: (1) Out-patient follow-up appointment.
(2) Drops to be used after discharge from the ward.

KERATOPLASTY (CORNEAL GRAFTING)

The nursing care of patients undergoing keratoplasty follows the principles of all intraocular operations. The graft can be a penetrating one i.e. the full thickness of the cornea, or a 'lamellar' which involves the replacement of only the superficial layers of the cornea.

The care of patients following penetrating keratoplasty varies from that of lamellar keratoplasty only in detail.

Pre-operative preparation is as for lens extraction except that the pupil must not be dilated, in fact most surgeons require the pupil to be constricted as an additional protection to the lens i.e. to prevent accidental trauma to the lens within a dilated pupil, and to prevent iris prolapse.

A 'Dunlopillo' or sorbo mattress is generally given to the patient as this is more comfortable for the long period of time that he will have to spend lying flat on his back, keeping as still as possible.

Sedation such as amylobarbitone or phenobarbitone 30 mg t.d.s. is often prescribed by the surgeon to discourage restlessness.

The operation is performed under a general anaesthetic and the patient prepared accordingly. Guttae pilocarpine 2% and guttae chloramphenicol 0·5% are instilled when the premedication is given.

Penetrating Keratoplasty

With this operation the surgeon penetrates the anterior chamber, therefore many of the complications that could occur with lens extraction are also possible.

The patient is returned to bed with both eyes padded and a Moorfields bandage applied. This is an extremely useful bandage because its wide double-thickness of material excludes light. The side tapes cross over behind the head to come up onto the forehead and are tied there over a cotton-wool swab. This will allow the bandage, when untied, to be turned up on the forehead without having to lift or move the patient's head. This bandage is ideal for use in keratoplasty and retinal detachment.

The dressing is usually left untouched for 48 hours and visitors are discouraged during this period. Toilet care is as for lens extraction.

1st Dressing

Follows the usual procedure for all intraocular dressings with additional observations:

1. Whether the graft is clear and in good position i.e. flush with the surrounding cornea.
2. That there is not an iris prolapse in the wound edges.
3. That all sutures are in place.
4. The condition of the anterior chamber. At the operation, the surgeon usually injects air into the anterior chamber to ensure that the wound is airtight, to keep the iris away from the cornea and thus to prevent the formation of anterior synechia. The size of the air bubble is noted; it will absorb slowly as the aqueous replaces it and the depth of the anterior chamber will thereafter be checked. It is extremely important that the patient should not squeeze his eye and thus prematurely squeeze out the air bubble.
5. The size and shape of the pupil is noted.

Should all be satisfactory, the pupil is fully dilated:

(a) As a prophylaxis against iritis and anterior synechia to the graft edges. The synechiae would only form if there was an aqueous leak.
(b) To prevent iris prolapse through the wound edges.

It is considered that the pupil is safely dilated should the edges appear under the wound because it is reasonable to suppose that with the application of the pad it will dilate out past the graft edges.

Oc. atropine 1% and oc. chloramphenicol 0·5% are instilled.

After the 1st Dressing, the patient is allowed to have the unoperated eye uncovered, a firm pad and bandage are applied to the operated eye. The patient is still nursed in the prone position with only one pillow.

As long as the eye remains satisfactory and comfortable, dressings are only done on alternate days. Should there be excessive lacrimation and the pad becomes wet and uncomfortable, it can be changed, provided the lids remain closed.

Complications

1. Iris prolapse, usually abscised by the surgeon.
2. Flat anterior chamber, dilatation and a very firm pad and bandage. If the chamber does not reform, the surgeon may inset additional sutures and inject an air bubble into the anterior chamber, or tighten the suture if a continuous one was used.
3. Anterior synechia may remain untreated or mydriasis and the application of a Maddox heater to enhance the absorption of the mydriatic.
4. Elevation of the graft, application of a pad and firm crepe bandage. If this is not effective and the elevation is very pronounced, the surgeon will often re-suture the elevated area.
5. Clouding or vascularization of the cornea, treated with local steroids such as

guttae prednisolone and often the addition of systemic steroids such as prednisolone 10–15 mg daily.

6th–7th day

1. The addition of oc. prednisolone to the dressing.

8th–9th day

1. Two extra pillows in a flat armchair position.

10th day

1. Dark glasses.
2. Guttae atropine 1% b.d.
   Guttae chloramphenicol 0·5% t.d.s.
   Guttae prednisolone 0·5% t.d.s.

11th day

1. Extra pillows with back-rest extended.

12th day

1. Up for bed-making.
2. Men may wear pyjamas.
3. Women may wear their own nightdresses.

13th day

1. The Sani-chair can be used.

14th day

1. Meals taken by bedside.
2. Men may be shaved.
3. Sutures may be removed.

15th day

1. Up with care.
2. General bath taken with pad and bandage applied.

21st day—DISCHARGE.

The patient is asked to wear his dark glasses whenever he is outdoors as the eye remains sensitive to light for several weeks while corneal sensation is impaired.

Guttae atropine 1% b.d.
Guttae prednisolone 0·5% t.d.s.

Lamellar Keratoplasty

Some surgeons only require the patient to be single padded following this operation. The regime is altered because there is no risk of iris prolapse, flat anterior chamber and anterior synechiae. The main complications that arise are elevation of the graft, vascularization of the cornea and opacification of the donor cornea.

This patient is usually allowed:

6th day

1. To sit up in bed.

7th day

1. Up for bed-making.

8th day

1. Meals by bed.

9th day

1. Up with care.

10th day

1. General bath.

11th day—DISCHARGE.

The dates for removal of the sutures vary from surgeon to surgeon, but may also depend upon:

1. The condition of the graft.
2. The type of sutures used.
3. The size of the graft.

When the sutures are removed, a pad and bandage is often applied for a period of 48 hours.

Give (1) Out-patient follow-up appointment.
(2) Drugs to be used after discharge from hospital.

RETINAL DETACHMENT

Detachment of the retina is generally treated as an ophthalmic emergency i.e. the patient is admitted to hospital as soon as the diagnosis is made and generally placed on bed rest before the operation within a few days.

Pre-operative Care

Admission

Although the patient may have come to hospital worrying about partial or even total visual loss, because the eye is not painful he rarely considers that his condition will turn out to be serious. It is therefore often something of a shock to him to be immediately admitted to hospital.

He is usually nursed in bed in a position corresponding to that of the detached retina. Not all surgeons require their patients to be 'positioned' and those who do are not generally insistent upon rigid positioning of the patient which sometimes necessitates blocking the foot of the bed and the use of sandbags to keep the head firmly in a set position. The main reason for positioning of the patient is to allow the retina to fall back into its natural position and for the sub-retinal fluid to absorb.

A conjunctival culture is taken and the eyelashes are cut. The patient is not usually double-padded at this stage, although some surgeons may require this after 24 hours. It is obviously far less worrying for the patient if he is allowed to keep his eyes uncovered and he will therefore be much more co-operative and less inclined to be restless. Occasionally, dark glasses are worn to discourage the patient from using his eyes too much i.e. reading, etc.

He is allowed a normal diet.

To encourage the patient to relax and to relieve the natural tendency to worry pre- and post-operatively, the surgeon usually prescribes a mild sedative such as phenobarbitone 30–60 mg t.d.s.

Prophylactic guttae chloramphenicol 0·5% is instilled to both eyes t.d.s. Full mydriasis is maintained in order that the surgeon can fully examine the fundus to determine the extent of the detachment, how many holes or tears may be present and the type of operative procedure to be adopted. At this stage, the surgeon generally makes a detailed drawing of the fundus which will be used as a guide during the operation.

Unlike many other types of operation, there is no set procedure for retinal detachment surgery and each case has to be treated on its own merits. For this reason, it is only possible to give a very broad outline of nursing care.

Basically, the type of operative procedure can be divided into:

1. Shortening procedure i.e. scleral resection or scleral overlay, with or without implant accompanied by the use of diathermy or cryo-therapy.
2. An encircling procedure, using a silicone strap and gutter rod or Arruga string.
3. Photocoagulation.

The nursing care of the shortening procedure can be compared with that for keratoplasty. Many surgeons require their patients to be positioned post-operatively and to remain on bed rest for 10 days to allow healing to take place. The patient may also remain double-padded for that period of time and be maintained on a soft diet to prevent excessive movement of the facial muscles and of course requires to be fed at all meals. Alternatively, surgeons may single-pad the patient after the first dressing and ambulate him on the 4–8th day allowing the patient to wear dark glasses.

Daily nursing care for shortening procedure:

1. 1st Dressing after 48 hours.
2. Visitors discouraged until after dressing.
3. No blanket bath until after 1st Dressing.
4. Sedation phenobarbitone 30–60 mg t.d.s.
5. Guttae atropine 1%
Oc. atropine 1% } daily
Oc. chloramphenicol 0·5% } daily
6. Daily dressings until 10th day.

7th day

Oc. prednisolone 0·5%.

10th day

1. Dark glasses may be worn.
2. Patient is allowed extra pillows if flat, armchair style.
3. Normal diet is resumed.
4. Men are allowed to be shaved.

5. Sedation is discontinued.
6. Conjunctival sutures are removed.
7. Guttae atropine 1% b.d.
   Guttae chloramphenicol 0·5% } t.d.s.
   Guttae prednisolone 0·5% }
8. Own night attire worn.

11th–12th day

1. Up for bed-making and long periods in a chair.
2. Use of Sani-chair.

13th day

Meals by bedside.

14th day

1. Up with care.
2. General bath taken.

21st day

Patient discharged.

During the period of ambulation, the patient is told not to stoop, to lift or carry anything heavy; this is again stressed on the patient's discharge from hospital. On occasions, patients have to change their occupation and engage in less strenuous work. This may present problems but with the aid of the Medical Social Worker a satisfactory alternative is generally found.

As in the nursing care of keratoplasty, it is very important to keep the patient relaxed and happy, to talk to him about current topics and to help him to pass the time with his radio and a 'talking book'; this is a machine which plays tape recordings of books read aloud. There is a large variety of books to choose from and one or two patients at one time can listen with head-phones or pillow-phones. A foam or Dunlopillo mattress is more comfortable for long periods of bed rest.

The Encircling procedure often consists of a strap and gutter or its equivalent being placed extraocularly, 10 mm or more posterior to the limbus, around the eye under the extrinsic muscles and then tightened. This has the effect of slightly compressing the eye and indenting the retina. The only sutures are those holding the strap in position and those in the conjunctiva. There is no reason for a prolonged period of bed rest, so the patient is generally allowed up after 2–3 days and gently ambulated. Frequently, discharge is on the 10th day.

STRABISMUS

The operation for correction of strabismus is an extraocular procedure, no incision is made into the eyeball, consequently this entails very little in the way of pre-operative preparation.

The majority of patients are children or young adults, although operations are performed upon older people.

Admission need not take place until twenty-four hours prior to operation and, for the young, this is a less traumatic experience than removing them from their home or school for a long period. The patient is examined by the orthoptist, either on the day of admission or the morning of operation, and another Orthoptic Report is completed for the surgeon.

It is essential to establish which eye is for operation, because this may not always be 'the squinting eye' and some parents or patients can be quite alarmed on being told that 'the good eye' is to be operated upon. The surgeon will already have explained the reason for this and reassured them.

A conjunctival culture is omitted and many surgeons do not require the eyelashes to be cut. Guttae chloramphenicol 0·5% is instilled into both eyes t.d.s. from admission.

On the Day of Operation

The patient is prepared as for general anaesthesia; although this operation can be performed on adults under local anaesthesia, this is rarely necessary.

Guttae chloramphenicol 0·5% and guttae Otrivine-Antistin, to whiten the eye, are instilled.

On return from theatre, the patient does not usually have his eye covered although, at a later period, babies sometimes need splinting of their arms to prevent rubbing of their eyes. The patient may be nursed in any position.

The following day the patient is allowed up without restriction. Guttae chloramphenicol 0·5% is instilled t.d.s., and oc. chloramphenicol nocte. No dressing is applied unless there is a tendency to rub the eye. A lint swab folded in half is sometimes attached by Sellotape just below the infraorbital margin should the eye water. In cases of severe lacrimation, a pad and bandage may be more comfortable for the patient.

The patient is encouraged to use his eyes as before, and, if he previously wore glasses, continues to do so. Reading, jig-saw puzzles, television, in fact any occupational therapy, are encouraged with children and young adults.

On the 3rd day post-operatively, the patient is seen by the surgeon and orthoptist, and providing no further surgery is required he is allowed home, back to school or work.

6/0 plain catgut is often used to sew up the conjunctiva, therefore there is no suture to remove.

Oculentum chloramphenicol 0·5% b.d. is usually prescribed for discharge.

Because of the comparative lack of intensive care to the eye and the short period of time required for hospital treatment, the operation for correction of squint may be considered to be a slight one or 'not very serious'; however, babies and young children who have squints may also have associated congenital abnormalities e.g. cardiac disorders. These conditions should have been previously diagnosed and supervised, but the nurse must always be particularly attentive to these young patients in the immediate post-operative period and also be aware of any dangers which could arise.

CARE AND STERILIZATION OF OPHTHALMIC INSTRUMENTS

Forceps

All forceps used in ophthalmic surgery are delicate precision-made instruments and must be handled with great care as they are easily damaged.

Before use, they should be carefully examined to make sure they are in perfect condition. The very fine toothed and non-toothed iris forceps may have to be examined with the aid of a loupe.

After use, they should be carefully washed with a soft toothbrush and dried before putting away, with metal or rubber bands holding the forceps closed to protect the ends.

Scissors

These should be tested before use by cutting a fine wisp of damp cotton wool. If the blades are not sharp they must be sent for repair. Particular attention should be paid to the tips of scissors, as they are very easily damaged. After use, scissors are carefully washed and dried. They should be stored hanging up, but if this is not possible, rubber tubing should be placed over the tips of sharp pointed scissors. De Weckers iris scissors are tested in the same way, but must be taken apart for cleaning and dried before being reassembled. They should be stored in velvet-lined boxes, but if these are not available, scissors should be kept closed in the same way as forceps.

Knives

All knives should be tested before use by placing on the open fingers of one hand and being allowed to slide onto the kid-skin of a drum held in the other hand; the point should pass through the skin under its own weight, and as the blade is withdrawn the skin should be cut by its entire length in order to test the cutting edge. Any knife which is not perfectly sharp either at the point or cutting edge must not be used, and must be sent for repair.

After use, a knife is cleaned by drawing the blade through a wet swab with cutting edge outwards, and then dried in the same way using a fine instrument cloth.

All knives should be stored in specially made velvet-lined boxes, and great care should be taken when removing or replacing a knife. The best method for removal is to press the handle with the thumb and then hold the knife just below the blade with the first two fingers of the same hand. In replacement, the handle should be lowered into the box first. A corneal trephine should be tested by turning on a kid drum. If the trephine is in good condition it should perforate the kid by its own weight.

After use, a trephine should be taken apart, cleaned and dried before reassembling. This is done by passing an orange stick, with wisps of wool twisted round it, hrough the lumen of the trephine from the blunt end. The trephine is stored in its own specially made box.

Sterilization

1. Dry heat
2. Steam
3. Boiling
4. Chemical solution or gas.

Dry heat is the method of choice whenever possible. The instruments are placed in metal boxes with the knives on special racks and baked at 150°C for two hours. Sutures, syringes, bowls and receivers may also be sterilized in this way.

Steam autoclaving is the best method for equipment which cannot be sterilized by dry heat e.g. diathermy leads, all rubber tubing and pipettes, etc. This method is also best for any instruments which may be required quickly as the entire process including sterilization and the restoration to atmospheric pressure from the vacuum is completed at 25 kg pressure and temperature 150°C in 2 minutes, or for 16 kg pressure at 150°C in 7 minutes.

If neither equipment is available it will be necessary to boil instruments. Distilled water must be used to prevent furring, and the instruments boiled for 5 minutes. In this case, knives and scissors must be sterilized in whichever chemical solution is advised by the hospital pathologist, but they must be immersed in boiling water for one minute before use, thus ensuring the removal of all traces of chemical.

In Ophthalmic Theatres, there is certain equipment which must not be subjected either to heat or moisture e.g. leads of cryosurgical units. These are sterilized by formalin vapour, although this method is now felt to be unsatisfactory and ethylene oxide gas is preferred whenever available.

GLOSSARY

Accommodation—The act of altering the focus of the eye so that divergent rays, coming from near objects are brought to a focus on the retina. The lens has the power to enable it to increase its convexity (and thus allow near objects to be focused).

Achromatopsia—Colour blindness.

Albino—A person with 'blonde' hair and 'pink' eyes, deficient in pigment—see choroid.

Amaurosis—A serious defect of vision.

Amblyopia—A defect of vision without any visible sign of disease.

Anterior chamber (A.C.)—The space posterior to the cornea and anterior to the iris, containing aqueous humour.

Aphakia—Absence of the lens.

Aqueous humour—A clear watery fluid resembling lymph, constantly being secreted by the ciliary processes of the uveal tract; it circulates in the A.C. and drains away via the angle (between the iris and the cornea) into the corneo-scleral filtration spaces, the minute circular canal of Schlemm, finally to reach the larger veins outside the eyeball.

Astigmatism—An irregular curvature of the cornea, resulting in the condition in which a point source of light cannot be brought to a focus upon the retina without the aid of a correcting lens.

Binocular vision—The ability to use both eyes together.

Blepharitis—Inflammation of the lid margins.

Bulbar Conjunctivitis—Inflammation of the conjunctiva covering the anterior third of the eyeball, from the corneo-scleral margin to the fornices.

Buphthalmos (Ox-eye)—General enlargement of the eyeball due to infantile glaucoma.

Canaliculi—The tear passages leading from the lacrimal puncta to the lacrimal sac.

Canthus—The angle formed at the junction of the upper and lower lids; the inner (medial) and outer (lateral).

Capsulotomy—Operation following 'extracapsular cataract extraction' involving the making of a hole in the posterior capsule of the lens.

Carbolization—The treating of a corneal ulcer with pure carbolic, usually applied with a sharpened orange stick.

Cartella—Protective eye shield.

Cataract—Opacity of the lens.

Chalazion—An enlargement of a Meibomian gland, the result of obstruction of the duct.

Chemosis—Oedema of the conjunctiva.

Choroid—The vascular lining of the eyeball forming the posterior third of the uveal tract, continuous anteriorly with the ciliary body. It contains pigment cells and blood vessels, giving it a dark brown colour. The pigment is absent in the albino.

Cryoextraction of lens—Low temperature lens removal.

Cycloplegics—Drugs used to dilate the pupil and paralyse the ciliary muscle.

Cilia—Eyelashes.

Cyclitis—Inflammation of the ciliary body.

Dacryoadenitis—Inflammation of the lacrimal gland.

Dacryocystitis—Inflammation of the lacrimal sac.

Dialysis, retinal—Peripheral tear of retina at ora serrata.

Diplopia—Double vision.

Discission—Operation for congenital cataract, or certain types of traumatic cataract, in which the anterior capsule is ruptured and the lens substance left to absorb, or later evacuated.

Ectropion—Eversion of the eyelid.

Entropion—Inversion of the eyelid.

Enucleation—Removal of the eye.

Epicanthus—A vertical fold of skin at the inner canthus.

Epiphora—Overflow of tears due to inadequate drainage.

Evisceration—Removal of the cornea and the contents of the eye within the sclera, necessitated by infection in the eyeball, without severing the optic nerve.

Exenteration of the orbit—Removal of eyelids and orbital contents.

Extracapsular extraction—Operation for cataract when the posterior lens capsule is left intact, the anterior capsule is opened and the lens contents evacuated.

Exophthalmos—(Proptosis) prominence of the eyeball.

Fornix—Where the bulbar conjunctiva is reflected onto the eyelid to meet the palpebral conjunctiva and forms a loose pouch. As this occurs at both upper and lower lids, there is therefore an upper and lower fornix.

Fundus—The interior of the back of the eye, which may be viewed with an ophthalmoscope.

Glaucoma—A condition of the eye in which the intraocular pressure is raised.

Hemianopia—Loss of half of the visual field.

Hordeolum—Stye.

Hypermetropia—Long sight.

Hyphaema—Blood in the anterior chamber.

Hypopyon—Cells in the A.C. due to pus or inflammation in the eyeball.

Iridectomy—Excision of a portion of iris.

Iridocyclitis—Inflammation of iris and ciliary body.

Iris abscission—Excision of iris.

Iris bombé—Ballooning forwards of the iris.

Iritis—Inflammation of the iris.

Keratitis—Inflammation of the cornea.

Keratic precipitates (K.P.)—Deposits from the uvea on the posterior surface of the cornea.

Keratoplasty—Operation performed to transplant an area of cornea from a donor eye to a recipient.

Keratoconus—Conical cornea, due to a gradual atrophic thinning.

Lacrimal apparatus—Consisting of the lacrimal glands, lacrimal puncta, the canaliculi, the lacrimal sac and the nasolacrimal duct, known as the tear apparatus.

Limbus—The corneo-scleral junction. The junction of the bulbar conjunctiva with the corneal epithelium.

Macropsia—The state in which objects appear to be larger than normal.

Macula lutea—The retinal area associated with greatest visual acuity, due to the concentration of cones situated 2 mm to the temporal side of the entrance of the optic nerve in the line of direct vision.

Maddox heater—Electric eye heater.

Meibomian cyst—See Chalazion.

Metamorphopsia—The state in which objects appear to be distorted.

Miotic—A drug which constricts the pupil.

Mydriasis—Dilatation of the pupil.

Mydriatic—A drug which dilates the pupil, but which is not a cycloplegic.

Myopia—Short sight.

Nystagmus—Disturbance of normal ocular posture consisting of quick involuntary oscillatory movements of the eye, usually in the horizontal direction and bilateral.

Ophthalmia Neonatorum—'Persistent discharge from the eyes of an infant commencing within 21 days of birth'. This is a notifiable condition.

Orthoptic treatment—Special exercises used in an endeavour to restore single binocular vision.

Palpebral conjunctiva—Conjunctiva lining the lids, which is reflected at the fornix to join the Bulbar Conjunctiva.

Panophthalmitis—Suppuration of the entire eyeball.

Papilla—Optic disc.

Papilloedema—Oedema of the optic disc not usually associated with any inflammatory change.

Paracentesis—Tapping of the anterior chamber to evacuate it.

Perimeter—An instrument used for measuring the visual field.

Photophobia—Dislike of light.

Polyopia—Is present when more than two images of an object are produced e.g. as in early cataract, and may be monocular or binocular.

Presbyopia—A state of insufficiency of accommodation due to advancing age.

Proptosis—See Exophthalmos.

Pterygium—A triangular fold of hyaline degeneration extending over the edge of the cornea, either medially or laterally, which may reach the pupillary area.

Ptosis—A drooping of the upper lid.

Recession—A muscle operation for squint when the muscle is cut from its insertion and re-attached more posteriorly.

Refraction—The testing of vision to estimate the degree, should it exist, of any refractive error.

Resection—A muscle operation for squint when a section of muscle is removed and the muscle re-attached at its original insertion.

Retina—The innermost, or nervous, coat of the eye, lying between the hyaloid membrane of the vitreous body and the choroid.

Retinoblastoma—Neuroepithelioma, glioma of the retina usually occurring in children under five years. Can be unilateral or bilateral, is considered to be congenital and possibly hereditary (a malignant tumour).

Retinoscopy—A 'shadow' test for the refraction of the eye, made by observing the movement of light and shadow within the pupil during reflection of light into the eye from a mirror.

Scotoma—A defect in the field of vision.

Strabismus—Squint, the upset in the balance of the co-ordination of the six pairs of extrinsic ocular muscles.

Symblepharon—The adhesion of the eyelid to the eyeball.

Synechia—(1) Anterior Synechia—The adhesion of the iris to the cornea.

(2) Posterior Synechia—The adhesion of the iris to the lens, its capsule or its substance, or to the vitreous.

Tarsorrhaphy—Suturing together of the lid margins, in total or part, resulting in their adhesion.

Tenotomy—Operation for squint involving the division or weakening of one of the extrinsic ocular muscles.

Trephine—Operation for glaucoma to produce artificial drainage of the aqueous humour through a 1·5–2 mm aperture made at the corneo-scleral margin, generally in the 12 o'clock meridian of the eyeball.

Trichiasis—An irregularity of the eyelashes which grow inwards towards the cornea causing irritation and ulceration of the cornea.

Uveitis—Inflammation of the uveal tract (comprising the iris, ciliary body and choroid).

Visual acuity—The acuity of vision, generally expressed by a fraction corresponding with a Test Type and the distance separating it from the patient.

Visual field—The area of visual awareness within which objects are seen when a patient is looking straight ahead at one fixed point.

Vitreous body—or Vitreous humour, a gelatinous transparent substance, varying in density, enclosed in the hyaloid membrane lying posterior to the lens.

Vitreous-rete mirabile—Vascular proliferation in vitreous.

INDEX